I loved the book, m~~ostly because it is filled~~ with writing
exercises inspired by spirituality and wisdom; and so
the exercises can have transcendent healing effects. *Heal
Your Self with Writing* pulls wisdom from all across
world civilizations—from Lao Tzu to a female Sufi
to Booker T. Washington to Steve Jobs. The writing is
smooth and so there is no heavy medicinal effect to the
healing. It feels more like healing with natural remedies.
It cleans the chakras. *Heal Your Self with Writing* is an
elixir for the soul.

> —George Davis, *Psychology Today*

This is so much more than a book on writing. It is a
guide to the soul's journey, with Catherine Ann Jones as
a compassionate teacher and wise companion along the
way.

> —Dr. Betty Sue Flowers,
> Series Consultant/Editor, *Joseph
> Campbell and the Power of Myth*

Heal Your Self with Writing is much more than a
"how-to" book. It is a spiritual manual of what it means
to live authentically, persuasively written, psychologi-
cally wise, and full of pertinent examples and exercises.
Catherine has been where she is talking about, drawing
on a lifetime of experiences and inner work. The result is
a marvelous fruit contributing totally to the new movement that sees art and healing as part of the same higher
and deeper purpose in the emerging culture of our time.

> —Jay Ramsay, *Crucible of Love: The
> Alchemy of Passionate Relationships*

I deeply value the soft voice of wisdom in this book. The accounts of encounters with shamans and mysterious teachers are unforgettable. On every page we find something to cherish: an exercise to stir the depths, a quotation to remember always, an insight to open the way. Catherine Ann Jones is a true friend to the soul.

—Dianne Skafte, Ph.D., *Listening to the Oracle*

Through a carefully designed sequence of examples and step-by-step writing exercises, Jones takes us on an informative journey of self-discovery and self-knowledge invaluable for care and healing of the soul, fascinating for anyone simply interested in exploring a deeper approach to life, and invaluable for anyone looking for healing.

—Selden Edwards, *New York Times* best-selling author of *The Little Book* and *The Lost Prince*

Through simple, anyone-can-do-them exercises, Jones makes plain the power of words to broaden your perspective, exorcise your demons, and yes, change your life for the better. It's a book that would have come in handy during my own dark nights of the soul, and I cherish it in happy times as its lessons brighten an already bright spirit.

—Matt R. Lohr, Co-author, *Dan O'Bannon's Guide to Screenplay Structure*

Catherine Ann Jones shares her unique but universal journey, traveling beside us as we grow more deeply acquainted with our individual and archetypal selves. She is a wise and congenial guide, illustrating each exercise with personal stories and epigrams from literature that explode from the page. This book provides keys for gaining oneself through writing—a Way for writers to follow for a lifetime.

> —Alfred Collins, Ph.D., *Fatherson: A Self Psychology of the Archetypal Masculine*

Writing provides its own form of the hero's journey. With Catherine Ann Jones as your guide, those who engage *Heal Your Self with Writing* will enter the most profound journey of all: into the depths of self-remembering to retrieve one's narrative identity.

> —Dennis Slattery, Ph.D., *Riting Myth, Mythic Writing: Plotting Your Personal Story*

One thing Catherine Ann Jones knows how to do is tell a story. Using examples from her own life, she shows how to use the stories people have inside themselves, and those they tell themselves about themselves, with the express purpose of healing themselves, transforming the hard rocks of life into jewels. Even if you're not a writer, this is a great book to help you get to know yourself better.

> —Amy Corzine, *The Secret Life of the Universe: The Quest for the Soul of Science*

Heal Your Self with Writing is a well-written—and useful—book for anyone wishing to explore the depths of their interior life and personal connections with the unseen and unspoken mysteries of existence. I highly recommend it to people of all ages.

—Arthur Kornhaber, M.D., Life Fellow, American Academy of Child and Adolescent Psychiatry, American Board of Psychiatry and Neurology, American Medical Association

Wonderful! Very practical exercises that can free us from past traumas and release our creative energies. Many of the exercises are not only therapeutic but also fun. Read, practice, and be healed. Then write a note to the author to thank her for a life-changing book.

—Ravi Ravindra, Ph.D., *The Spiritual Roots of Yoga*

Heal Your Self with Writing is insightful and wise, tender and true. Catherine Ann Jones reminds us, "Ultimately, we long for what we truly are." Her writing will bring you back to who you are and help you trust your deepest knowing. For whatever's unhealed, open this book and read, then turn to your journal and write. You'll be so glad you did!

—Patrice Vecchione, *Writing and the Spiritual Life: Finding Your Voice by Looking Within*

Catherine Ann Jones is dedicated to the healing power of writing. In this book she shows you how you too can use writing to release old fears, pain, and conditioning so that you are finally free to live your life fully and happily.

—Marilyn Tam, *The Happiness Choice*

Heal Your Self with Writing shows how we can engage in deep inner work through writing. The use of focused journaling helps us take ownership of our full lifespan and find healing possibilities in all that has happened to us, nothing left out or unappreciated.

—David Richo, Ph.D.,
How to Be an Adult in Love

In this treasure of a book, *Heal Your Self with Writing*, Catherine Ann Jones explores the idea of how we can change the stories that we tell ourselves from our past that are holding us back and learn how to heal them through writing. By doing this, we can bring our world back into balance and create the life that we want from a stronger place of truth, awareness, and connectedness.

—Jen Grisanti, *Change Your Story,
Change Your Life: A Path to Success*

Using proven exercises from her workshop bearing the same name, Jones provides a worthy guidebook where a writer can find therapeutic release through the writing process.

—Kathie Fong Yoneda, *The Script-Selling
Game: A Hollywood Insider's Look At
Getting Your Script Sold and Produced*

Like *The Way of Story*, the author's previous work, *Heal Your Self with Writing* is a testament to the healing power of narrative and story, which connect us to the soul. I'm sure that the emotional resonance produced by writing in response to the exercises in this book will clarify the reader's values, improve self-understanding, relieve stress, and generally inform the reader of his or her internal state of affairs.

—Lionel Corbett, M.D., *The Sacred Cauldron: Psychotherapy as a Spiritual Practice*

A must-read for anyone who feels mired in an old life script and longs for the creative freedom of new perspectives. Reading *Heal Your Self with Writing* is like opening a treasure chest of alchemical exercises and wisdom that reveals the gold in the depth of personal memories. A book to be turned to again and again.

—Hendrika de Vries, Marriage and Family Therapist

For *The Way of Story: The Craft and Soul of Writing*:

Catherine Ann Jones's focus, clarity, and gentle but spot-on reactions help identify the weak or lazy spots in your writing. Thank God! She is the elevator of purpose.
—Joan Buck, *Vanity Fair*

A safe place in which to discover oneself as a writer. Great exercises which open up a deeper process while learning the essential steps of story structure.

—Linda Leonard, Jungian Analyst and Author, *Wounded Woman: Healing the Father-Daughter Relationship*

The Way of Story invigorated my work in a special way. Catherine is a writer's writer and a gifted teacher.

—Barry J. Mills, M.D., Ph.D., Santa Barbara, CA

I took your Way of Story workshop four years ago at Esalen Institute, but was not yet ready for your course then. Later I bought *The Way of Story* book and it has been my guiding light in writing my memoir. I'm sending you a copy of my book with a dedication to you in gratitude for what you have taught me. Thank you again for your brilliant guiding light in my life.

—Meg Robinson, UK, *Drawn by a Star: Adventures in Patagonia*

Catherine Ann Jones showed me how to write my way out of the darkness and into the light.

—Beth T., Athens, GA

Catherine Ann Jones is a superb teacher and a writer who knows how to open doors to the creative, psychological, and spiritual. A brilliant being!

—Marietta S., San Francisco, CA

Wonderful!! Absolutely amazingly, delightful! Catherine knows how to break through your barriers and tap into your own personal creative potential. She is gentle, while prodding your brain to open up.

—Mieke Blom, The Netherlands

Your structure gave my story wings. I've never been so clear on what I want to write.

—Linda L., Ann Arbor, MI

Catherine Ann Jones is a clear, compassionate soul who gives her students exercises that are pathways to their own souls. This work is about so much more than writing. As you work the process, you realize that this experience will continue to inform your writing as well as your whole life. So many seeds were given that I expect to be picking from this writing garden for the rest of my life.

—Cynthia C., Bethlehem, IN

Heal Your Self
WITH
Writing

Catherine Ann Jones

DIVINE
ARTS

Published by DIVINE ARTS
DivineArtsMedia.com

An imprint of Michael Wiese Productions
12400 Ventura Blvd. # 1111
Studio City, CA 91604
(818) 379-8799, (818) 986-3408 (Fax)
www.mwp.com

Cover design by Johnny Ink www.johnnyink.com
Copyediting by Gary Sunshine
Book layout by Gina Mansfield Design

Printed by McNaughton & Gunn, Inc., Saline, Michigan
Manufactured in the United States of America

Library of Congress Cataloging-in-Publication Data

Jones, Catherine Ann, 1944-
 Heal your self with writing / Catherine Ann Jones.
    pages cm
 ISBN 978-1-61125-016-9 (pbk.)
 1. Diaries--Therapeutic use. 2. Self-actualization (Psychology) 3. Authorship-
-Psychological aspects. 4. Self-help techniques. I. Title.
 RC489.D5J66 2013
 616.89'165--dc23
                                   2013007151

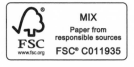

FSC
www.fsc.org

MIX
Paper from
responsible sources
FSC® C011935

Printed on recycled stock.
Publisher plants ten trees for every one tree used to produce this book.

for Sri Adwayananda

———•———

Waves are nothing but water.
So is the sea.
~ Sri Atmananda

Table of Contents

Author's Note

Writing is a solitary act. One of the great rewards of writing this book has been to learn that I am not alone and that I do get by with the help of my friends.

Special thanks to my first and constant reader, my son, Christopher R. Rao, who believed in me back when, for his enthusiasm and keen eye; to Dr. Dianne Skafte for her perceptive comments and continuous support; and to Dr. Betty Sue Flowers for her sharp editorial skills and longtime friendship.

Appreciation is also due to my publishers, Michael Wiese and Manny Otto, and editor Gary Sunshine for his insistence on clarity. Thanks also to the entire team at Michael Wiese Productions, who helped to shepherd this project through the web of publication and release. It takes a village to make a book.

And finally, I feel a special gratitude toward my many students and clients both here and abroad who over the years have enabled me to learn while teaching them.

Introduction

It's all right, it's over. It's just a memory.
J. K. Rowling, *Harry Potter and the Chamber of Secrets*

Our lives may be determined less by past events than by the way we remember them. If we learn how to reframe the pieces of our past and re-vision our life story so that suffering becomes meaningful, we can radically boost our chances of healing, empowerment, growth, and transformation. Focused journaling — short writing exercises designed to facilitate self-healing — is an extremely powerful tool to achieve this aim.

Expressing and listening to one's story is an ancient mode of healing. There is an overwhelming need today for people to be heard, to tell their stories, to learn and grow from their experience both individually and collectively. It is crucial that we offer constructive and transformative methodology for this process. It may mean the difference between deep, transformative healing and some form of "acting out" or self-destruction — both personally and collectively.

My first book, *The Way of Story: The Craft and Soul of Writing*, is for creative writers of all forms of narrative (plays, screenplays, fiction, and nonfiction including memoir). It began as a series of workshops for creative writers, and these workshops in some way mirrored my lifelong journey from actor to playwright to screenwriter to professor. *The Way of Story* uses short exercises to illustrate and develop self-understanding and also sometimes incorporates elements of memoir, i.e., examples and insights from my own life's journey. Teaching these workshops for over three decades now, I have seen hundreds of students perfect their craft by using highly personal, traumatic events as a catalyst for creative expression. Yet during the process of perfecting their writing craft, something else occurred. Many of these participants shared with me how the workshop experience unexpectedly helped them to break free of the trauma itself — even after many years. Witnessing these dramatic personal triumphs firsthand inspired me to teach workshops to both writers and non-writers as a catalyst in order that the primal creative process could heal as well as instruct. Not just to understand the psychology of the trauma and suffering, but to transform the pain and the memory of the pain itself. Again, I was enriched and humbled to see the participants in these workshops transform their personal demons and deepen their own life journey toward balance and wholeness.

During a twenty-year period teaching graduate school first in New York at The New School and later at the University of Southern California in Los Angeles, I discovered the value of using short writing exercises to quickly teach certain principles. I also studied ancient shamanic practices during a Fulbright research year in India, which has stimulated certain alternative approaches in my work. Later on, I went back to school for a graduate degree in Depth Psychology and Archetypal Mythology, and now consciously incorporate an understanding of psychological processes into my teaching and writing, as well.

The culmination of all these experiences has led organically to the book you are holding now.

I first taught *Heal Your Self with Writing (Healing Trauma Through Writing)* as a seminar at the Esalen Institute in Big Sur, California, several years ago, and was amazed at the response. Several participants felt that they were able to heal a split within themselves that had not been healed with years of traditional therapy. One woman later wrote to me that she had felt separated from herself since being victimized by a sexual assault at the age of fifteen. After the Esalen experiential workshop, she felt reconnected to both her body and her mind through the focused journaling exercises. She later wrote to me that she had "returned to herself."

What had occurred in this short period of time to achieve this life-changing result? One thing was crystal clear. I was not the cause, only the catalyst. She had herself done the inner work necessary to heal the split within, and she had done this through specific writing exercises combined with a fierce courage and resolve to change.

We all know the value of psychology in uncovering our deepest feelings, and the importance of catharsis in temporarily releasing our pain. Yet while psychological techniques may help prepare us for the magical journey of healing, they sometimes are not enough to lead us through the deeper journey of transformation. Catharsis without transcendence risks reliving negative patterns over and over, even reinforcing them, rather than truly putting them behind us.

What psychology does well is help us understand how we feel. What traditional psychology doesn't always do is provide the way through. Einstein remarked that you can never discover a solution on the same level as the problem. Similarly, only by rising to a higher level of consciousness can an ultimate solution to psychological problems be found. Healing and transformation are possible only through changing one's perspective from within.

There is a Native American parable about a grandfather who says to his grandson, "I feel as if I have two wolves fighting in my heart. One wolf is vengeful and angry; the other is loving and compassionate." When his grandson asks him which wolf will win the fight in his heart, the old man replies, "The one I feed."

How do we learn to "feed" the stories that heal? How do we put together the pieces of our past? How can we re-vision our life story so that pain becomes meaningful and actually promotes growth and transformation?

Heal Your Self with Writing offers a step-by-step journey of discovery and re-visioning through focused journaling. This serves as a basic survival safeguard and adds to global health by offering a creative tool for individuals, therapists, and teachers in dealing with grief and trauma in today's world as well as providing a means for deeper self-inquiry. In this way, global healing takes place one individual, one tribe at a time.

Telling stories about our past through this approach can help change our perspectives, enabling both healing and empowerment. In this way, we are able to make meaning out of memory and put the past where it belongs — behind us.

If it is time to heal the past and glean meaning from what you have experienced, this book may serve. If you are a creative person looking for an inspired way to live your life or someone who long ago laid aside your dream of creating and feel instinctively that it is time to recover the creative within, read on. Or if you are someone who has been a professional creative yet seeks to replenish the well, needing a stimulus to pick up the pen or brush, this book may serve as a catalyst to return home, an invitation to the muse, a bridge back to your creativity and Self.

Writing has been, for me, the greatest therapy I know. It is my hope that this book and its exercises will provide the same for you.

Catherine Ann Jones
Ojai, CA
June 15, 2013

Chapter One

What Story
Are You Living?

———

To be a person is to have a story to tell.
Isak Dinesen

An only child, I began at age twelve writing in journals. The journal became my best friend, my confidante, and sent me on a path of self-discovery. Later, earning my living as an actor and then as a playwright in New York City, followed by a career as a television writer and screenwriter in Hollywood, I experienced writing as a way of understanding not only myself, but also the world and others.

What is the first thing that pops into your mind when you read this sentence: "Whose life are you living?" Jot it down. Home is where our stories begin, so let's first explore our family of origin.

Sometimes we assume we are living our life when instead we are living the life a parent or spouse expects of us. Is this so with you?

Nothing has a stronger influence on children
than the unlived life of the parents.
C. G. Jung

The exercises presented throughout this book are designed either for groups — classroom or personally organized weekly groups — or for individuals. For groups, I suggest a time for writing of five to ten minutes depending on the nature of the exercise. For individuals, allow the freedom to take as long as necessary.

EXERCISE

Are you living the life your father or mother expected you to live? Identify a time in your life when you gave up your own story to live — even for a short time — for the expectations of another. Write about this and how it felt.

Of course, it may not always be a parent's influence. We may be living a life based on someone else, someone we admire and wish to be like. It might be a highly respected teacher or mentor, or even a public icon we've never actually met. There is another internal pressure, sometimes subtle and unspoken, sometimes not. This is the pressure to achieve — or not achieve — something desired by either parent or other, and not fulfilled by them in their lives. Either may cause the same block. For instance, a parent may outwardly seem to encourage the child to succeed, yet inwardly, unconsciously, be envious of his or her own child's success.

EXERCISE

- Consider some dream or goal one of your parents desired yet did not achieve. Write about that.

- Now zero in on either a felt pressure to achieve this goal on behalf of his or her parent or an understanding not to surpass that parent in fulfilling this goal. And write about this.

- Finally, ask yourself whether you are now living your dream or your parent's.

> *Don't live someone else's life.*
> *Don't be trapped by dogma — which is*
> *living with the results of other people's*
> *thinking. And most important, have the*
> *courage to follow your heart and intuition.*
> *Everything else is secondary.*
> Steve Jobs

Remember we are here to grow and evolve toward wholeness. It is all process — the process of soul evolution.

How can you know if you are living the life you are meant to live? How can you know yourself? The stories we tell ourselves determine to a great extent who we appear to be to others — and often even to ourselves. Authenticity is crucial in the path to healing and to self-discovery. The stories we tell ourselves become who we are.

Whose Life Are You Living?

EXERCISE

Which components of your life have met your parents' expectations? And which have not met them?

Storytelling is not only the root of film, theatre, literature, and culture, but of the life experience itself. The listener or viewer maintains touch with his mythic Self and the truths there represented. In losing touch with our myths, there may be a danger of losing touch with ourselves.

Today, in modern life, a fragmentation separates most of us from our central core or soul. With all our outer progress, perhaps something has been lost which earlier cultures knew to value: the soul connection. What story do you choose to live by? The answer offers a clue to your soul, your deepest Self.

After having some success as a playwright in New York, I applied for and won a Fulbright research grant to study shamanic forms of storytelling in India. I wanted to go where story was more than entertainment, where it carried some deeper meaning and purpose. So for a year, I explored five-thousand-year-old shamanic rituals and dramatic forms in south India.

For thirty thousand years and in the earliest forms of oral tradition, shamans have tended the soul. The very word, *shaman*, coming from the Tungus people of Siberia, means "excited, moved, raised." The shaman journeys out of body to a realm beyond time and space. His soul leaves his body in trance state and travels to the underworld or skyward, returning with a message for the community. In this way, the shaman becomes a bridge between the two worlds of earth and spirit. The shaman is an ear for his community. He discovers where their suffering lies, and speaks to that.

What has this to do with us today? Since the Industrial Revolution, we have been split off from spirit. The price of outer, industrial success removed us from our connection to the land and its spirit. It vastly increased the pace of life, thereby affecting our quality of life and personal relationships. It replaced value on family and health with monetary value. It lessened our instinctive responses and gave us instead mental development. It created a greater distance from our soul. Today's Age of Information is a poor substitute for the callings of spirit. Information is not — nor ever was — wisdom. Knowledge is more than the naming of names, and survival more than material sustenance. In olden times a shaman would interpret psychological illness as a separation from soul. His job then was to retrieve the severed soul and unite or return it to the one possessed or ill.

In F. Scott Fitzgerald's classic novel, *The Great Gatsby*, Jay Gatsby illustrates the rags-to-riches American dream that gained prominence after we won the first World War. A self-made man, Jay Gatsby becomes a very wealthy man only to realize later that all he really wanted was the love of his childhood sweetheart, Daisy.

What we believe shapes who we are — even what we do or don't do. Let's look back and remember what we believed in our early years.

EXERCISE

At age 12, I believed _____

At age 22, I believed _____

At age 32, I believed _____

At age 42, I believed _____

Today I believe _____

Notice how what you thought to be true has changed over the years. Though there is continuity to your deeper Self, the personality and what it believes may change over the years — even drastically change.

It is crucial to ascertain what needs to change and what needs to remain constant, such as our core values, as these are the inner beacon of our outer journey.

EXERCISE

Focus on what about you has remained the same. Write a few lines about that. Look within. What has not changed over the years, what has remained constant?

Sometimes to discard one belief or identity for another is dramatic and may hurt others. To be authentic may sometimes appear ruthless, and, at first, may seem selfish. However, it is my experience that to be true to what one is, is kinder in the long run. For, in the end, to live a lie can hurt others more.

> *Two roads diverged in a wood,*
> *And I took the one less traveled by,*
> *And that has made all the difference.*
>   Robert Frost

Paul Gauguin was married with five children and working as a stockbroker and businessman when he became depressed and even attempted suicide. He was not living an authentic life. So he chose to radically change his life. He left his lucrative job and his family, and ended up painting in Tahiti, and the rest is history.

During my years in India, I was struck by the concept of *dharma*. In Sanskrit, dharma means "law" or "order." Dharma is the law of your existence or your true inner calling, and is much more than a job or vocation. It is said that to follow dharma wholeheartedly will invite invisible allies to come to your aid and support. It is written in ancient texts that it is better to be a good sweeper than a bad king — if being a sweeper is your dharma. So when we turn within to feel what our dharma is, it is vital to be honest about what stirrings are there. For instance, I know a remarkable woman who was a successful corporate lawyer, and not happy. She went back to school and became an elementary school teacher. Last year, she won a teaching award for the State of Washington, and remains passionate about teaching children!

Achieve goals that are truly appropriate for you and your soul's growth.

EXERCISE

Describe a time in your life when you followed your inner calling or dharma though it demanded some form of sacrifice.

In my years as a freelance writer in New York and later in Hollywood, I found this to be totally true. This is not to say it is always an easy path but certainly a fulfilling one. And there often seems to be some power at work to take care of those who follow their bliss. To honor what is deepest in one's Self is what ultimately matters. This means to dedicate yourself to achieve those goals that are most appropriate for you and your soul's growth. This has nothing to do with fame or money, but rather what is your soul's bidding, what will enable the soul to grow.

In *Hamlet*, Polonius speaks to his son who is going off to college:

This above all: to thine own self be true, And it must follow, as the night the day, Thou canst not then be false to any man. Farewell, my blessing season this in thee!
William Shakespeare

The first and foremost step is to accept who you are. Everything else follows. Your limitations are not set by who you are but rather who you think you're not. The people who are put in high regard and given much respect are those who are confident enough to believe in themselves. And it is far easier to believe in yourself if you are being an authentic Self.

Here's another thing. Sometimes we don't wish to be ourselves because we are all too aware of our faults. It is odd but sometimes a seeming fault in one's self can be a portal of discovery. Here's an example from history:

Sir Alexander Fleming discovered penicillin, the first antibiotic, in 1929, and in doing so, saved millions of lives. By 1927, Fleming was already well known from earlier work, and had developed a reputation as a brilliant researcher, but his laboratory was often untidy. This was always a fault he had: messiness. On September 3, 1928, Fleming returned to his laboratory having spent August on holiday with his family. Before leaving, he had messily stacked all his cultures of staphylococci together on a bench in a corner of his laboratory. On returning, Fleming noticed that one culture was contaminated with a fungus, and that the colonies of staphylococci that had immediately surrounded it had been destroyed, whereas other colonies farther away were normal. Fleming grew the mold in a pure culture and found that it produced a substance that killed a number of disease-causing bacteria. He identified the mold as being from the penicillium genus, and, after some months of calling it "mold juice," on March 7, 1929, he named the substance it released "penicillin." If he had been less untidy, this discovery may never have happened!

Negative Patterns

Negative patterns sometimes evolve for a reason. A child growing up in an alcoholic and/or abusive environment may create a wall around himself for protection. Such defensive methods may actually ensure surviving emotionally and physically through challenging and threatening times in our lives. Years pass, however, and though we are now safe, these walls and other defense mechanisms may sometimes sabotage both our personal and professional lives. The wall is no longer needed yet it remains. It has become habitual. The first step is to become aware of what we have built around us, and how this invisible wall prevents connecting and leading a full and meaningful life.

What stories do we tell ourselves to fortify the wall? Stories from the past live on in us long after the cause or effect is gone. *What you remember remembers you.* What we hold in our memory shapes both our present and future. Here's one example.

I recently taught *The Way of Story* workshop at the Esalen Institute in Big Sur, California. A woman had broken up with a man who also happened to be taking the workshop at the same time. Sitting in the circle across from a former lover made the woman increasingly uncomfortable. And though she had looked forward to taking the workshop, she now felt completely unable to focus. I spoke with her privately for a few minutes then asked if she could for a moment separate the perception of the man from the inner story she was telling and re-telling within. She closed her eyes and was soon able to discriminate between seeing him and listening to the story she was keeping alive within herself. I asked her, "So who is telling the story?" She laughed, took a deep breath, and was able to release the old track from her mind — at least enough to return and focus on the remaining days of the workshop. This is not to say that her work was done in this brief moment, but she had acquired a new tool in lessening the traumatic memory she had experienced from the breakup with her partner. With a small shift in perspective, she had gained an insight into a deeper Self, enabling her to step back and witness a life event that had stalled her moving forward into a new life.

So what exactly happened here? A woman felt powerless because she was unable to let go of a story she was holding on to which made her a victim. Even though she no longer saw this man, her former lover, she carried him within, and over and over again was keeping this victim version of her story alive. Thus, in doing so, she made herself more and more powerless. All she did now was step back and take responsibility for the story she was telling and re-telling. In undergoing this shift in perspective, she was able to see herself as separate from what she was doing. Thus, she became a witness to her own creation of her daily life. Isn't the power of the mind awesome?

EXERCISE

—•—

- Think of a difficult event or person from your past.

- Feel within the emotions associated with this event or person.

- Now visualize looking back across time and observe yourself telling the old story.

- Choose a perspective from where you stand now — one more acceptable.

- Write it down from this new perspective.

Choose Your Thoughts

As we grow, these negative, protective patterns may outlive their use. Then as maturity comes, we seek to create new, healthier patterns. It's not that the negative patterns leave altogether. They simply go dormant while the new, healthier patterns take over, as it were. We learn, as the old grandfather did, to feed the good wolf. It makes sense to accept this and to have compassion not only for the old negative patterns, which remain part of us in our life journey, but for the child or young adult who needed them at the time. Judging ourselves only adds weight to the unnecessary baggage we already carry.

Only when old patterns that no longer serve are released can new ones emerge. Sometimes, too, new, healthier habits must be in place before releasing the old ones.

When traumatic or disturbing events — either personal or collective — happen to us when young, we may not have possessed the words then to speak out. The words come later as we look squarely at our own lives and the world we live in, and at how we got here from there.

That which is unspoken becomes unspeakable.
Adrienne Rich, poet

Personal events are not the only forces that darken our psyches. Sometimes the soul's way is diametrically opposed to the collective tune, and we must find the courage to march to our own drum. A dramatic example from history is the brave souls who hid Jews during the time of Hitler and WWII. They chose, at considerable peril, to resist the collective rule and follow what they felt to be right. It is possible, peacefully, to separate yourself from the dysfunctional collective whose message is that we are helpless and must accept the world as it is, that we are powerless either to change it or our own lives. Consider this. If we wait for only the perfect people to change the world, it may be too late. If speaking out can help one other person, can we remain silent? How can I make a difference, be it ever so small? How do I choose to spend my free time? As Gandhi said, "Become the change you wish to see." Of course, this takes tremendous courage — both physically and morally. Without courage, change is seldom possible.

One isn't necessarily born with courage,
but one is born with potential. Without
courage, we cannot practice any other
virtue with consistency.

Maya Angelou

To be most effective, it is best if the movement toward change arises from within, that deeper part of our being. There is no greater force than being true to one's Self and finding the courage to move forward in a centered way. How many times have allies — visible and invisible — come to our aid when we walk our true walk?

Writing for the popular television series, *Touched by an Angel*, I learned how important it is to tell the story from the character's point of view or perspective. It is so in life as well. How we see our past is how our present will be imprinted. All we have are our thoughts, feelings, and sensations. These are what we remember; these become the memories — both good and bad — that constitute a life. How we view our life matters tremendously. If we go deep enough, have the courage to let go of the negative past, and allow a shift to occur away from those negative patterns that imprison us by recreating a habitual pattern of negative feelings and events, we can free ourselves.

When I am asked to present a talk or teach a writing workshop, I often state that those who wish to be writers and are not from a dysfunctional family background, I am sorry for you. There's no greater background for an artist than a dysfunctional family! Every time there is a terrific response of recognition and laughter.

The point is to use what you are given, and not let it use or destroy you. If we open and choose to change, it is possible. It is always possible.

Here's an example of a shift in seeing. Something occurs with a family member, friend, or business associate that causes us to become frustrated. You might habitually pronounce, "I'm frustrated." In this way, you become identified with frustration. You are walking frustration. Develop a practice of stepping back for a moment. Count to ten. Count to a hundred. Then just become aware of the frustration — without judgment or resistance. Instead of saying to yourself or others, "I am frustrated," try saying instead, "Frustration is there." See it as something separate from you, as an uninvited guest who has dropped by. In this way, perceiving a negative emotion as something separate can lessen its power. Remember you can only govern your reaction to what happens to you — not to what actually happens.

EXERCISE

Write and share a time in your life when instead of remaining in a negative response to something unpleasant, you stepped back and saw the incident or event from an entirely different perspective. What was different? Compare how you felt then and now.

Another tool that can be helpful is to develop a mental habit of shifting focus. When difficult times arise, refuse to stay with hurt, anger, and pain, and choose to focus instead on "What is the solution to this problem?" Doing this creates a spontaneous shift from a passive to an active focus.

EXERCISE

Think of a specific problem you are experiencing at this time in your life for which you blame someone else for its cause. It may be a weighty problem of relationship or finance or whatever. Attempt to shift your focus from what this person or problem is doing to you to "What can I do?" Make sure to focus on what you can do — not what someone else must do.

Of course, sometimes there does not seem a solution or way to fix a problem. Then, all we can do is to let it go. Yet there is one thing you can do to salvage something of value from even the most awful situation. As often as I can, after an unpleasant event, I simply shift my perspective from "What is happening to me?" to "What can I learn from this?" Somehow this simple shift in perspective can make all the difference. To learn is to grow, and it feels good to grow.

EXERCISE

Remember an unpleasant event from the past, one you have spent considerable time remembering and feeling bad about. Now ask yourself, "What did I learn from this?" or "What can I learn from this?" Write it down.

> *Life is a succession of lessons which must be lived to be understood.*
> Helen Keller

Everyone knows the amazing story of Helen Keller, an angry, lonely child who could not hear, speak, or see. She was a bright, passionate being locked inside until a remarkable teacher, Annie Sullivan, appeared to open the door. Helen Keller was not only required to make a great emotional shift within but to think outside the box. It was not easy for her or for her teacher, but they persevered and look at what happened! So when Helen Keller tells us — for she learned how to communicate — that life is a succession of lessons which must be lived to be understood, we are amazed and listen. It is pretty evident that without her devoted teacher, Annie Sullivan, who refused to accept failure, Helen Keller might never have uttered her first word, "Water." (See *The Miracle Worker,* the splendid film directed by Arthur Penn.)

EXERCISE

Recall a moment in your life when a teacher or mentor made all the difference. Write about the person who provided insight at a time you needed it most. Remember also to express your gratitude.

Re-visioning Your Life Story

When it is time for the old ways to leave us, it often feels like a kind of death, an ending of something. And yet, growth sometimes demands such endings. It may be a death of innocence, an end to a close relationship, a physical death of a loved one, or many other variations. This not only changes our outer life but alters the way we see ourselves and the world. Remember that how we see is essentially who we are.

> *...the sound of story is the*
> *dominant sound of our lives.*
> Reynolds Price

There is a wonderful true story of Nan-in, a Zen Master in the nineteenth century in Japan. A university professor had come to the Zen Master to inquire about Zen. As Nan-in served tea, he did a very odd thing. He kept pouring the tea after the cup was full.

The professor noticed the overflowing cup and exclaimed, "It is overfull. No more will go in!" Then the

Zen Master replied, "As you are full of your own opinions. How can I show you Zen unless you first empty your cup?"

So when there are endings in our life, we must let go, and empty our cup. If not, there is no place for the new. If you are not prepared to die daily, you will never live.

EXERCISE

Sit quietly for a few minutes with closed eyes. Take three deep breaths, and as you release each breath, let go of everything. Yes, everything. Then turn inward and ask, "What can I empty from my cup and what is preventing my doing it right now?"

Write down your responses to these questions. Be as honest as you dare. Know that it may be necessary to completely re-vision your life and who you are.

Courage is resistance to fear,
mastery of fear, not absence of fear.
Mark Twain

While we may not always have control over everything in our lives, we do have the power to face squarely what serves and what does not serve in our own evolution. By visualizing what we would like our future to look like, we lay the groundwork for things to come, which allows us to have a better idea of what we need to do, and how we should live our lives in order to achieve our goals.

Remember, too, that there is no action without choice.

> *Fate leads those who are willing.*
> Latin epigram

When we are centered in who we truly are deep down, there is less necessity to defend ourselves. What if we adopted a welcoming attitude to life, letting go of a habitual defensive or controlling attitude? What would we attract then? How might our life change?

Chapter Two

Why I Want
What I Can't Have

---

*The lamps are different but the Light
is the same.*
  Rumi

Can you remember wanting something so badly
that though it was never given, the desire or attraction
never left? Then years later, as an adult, you came across
that thing you so desired when young, and bought it for
yourself? I do.

Every single year, my mother would take me to the
downtown store and buy for me brand new black patent
leather shoes. When I was six years old, I saw *The Wiz-
ard of Oz.* So that year, I desperately wanted red shoes
like Dorothy. I didn't get them. I never got them. Black
shoes were more practical. Then, in my mid-twenties, I
happened to be passing a shoe store on Fifth Avenue in
New York City, and caught a glimpse of red shoes. Well, I
simply had to have them. I didn't need them, but I would
have them. After they were mine, it was wonderful — for
a few days. And then, somehow it didn't matter.

What had happened here? The desire — though
now unconscious most of the time — had lived on. And

probably when in my adult life something was missing, I glimpsed the red shoes, the unfulfilled childhood desire. And yet, after the first flush of owning and wearing them wore off, they no longer made me happy. The desire nature is strong in all of us, and yet if the first object we desire is fulfilled, it should always make us happy. Of course, it never does. If we cannot be happy in the moment, we will never be happy. The objects of desire are transient, ever changing. And temporary happiness is not an absolute. Let's examine then this process called desire.

Tell me what a man or woman desires and I will tell you who he or she is. As a deeper exploration of "what story are we living," it is important to look at what we desire.

The Nature of Desire

When we desire something intensely, the mind is restless, never still. It drives us on until we attempt to get what we want. Yet later on, even after achieving that desired object, sooner or later, we desire something else and the process repeats itself all over again. The question then is what will make us permanently happy? If the desired object does not bring happiness, then what does?

Here's what actually happens. When we achieve the object we desire, the mind becomes still, at peace. At this moment, happiness is experienced. So perhaps a shortcut to achieving happiness would be to find a way to still the restless mind. Not easily done, but certainly the right yellow brick road.

Now, of course, objects may be either material/concrete, human, or subtle. We identify with what we have. Who I am is what I own or what I have accomplished. For instance, having experienced fame for a time can become a subtle object we wish to possess again. Or it might be another's fame we covet. Or that person's spouse, or home. Endlessly comparing what I have with what the other has is a no-win game. And yet, we continually buy into the old adage that "The grass is greener on the other side of the fence." Why?

Then, too, sometimes the process is in identifying what we don't want, what doesn't fit or align with who we authentically are. Only after knowing what we don't want can we begin to discover what we do want. One thing is sure though. The more we can live in alignment with what we truly are, the easier it will become to let go of what prevents us from going forward.

There is probably more than one reason why we do what we do. Citing one cause for every effect is not very intelligent — it's rather like saying the cure of every illness is apple cider vinegar. Life is more complex than that — and, alas, so are we.

The Undercurrents of Desire

Sometimes, knowingly or unknowingly, we may be living out the unacknowledged dreams of our parents — wanting to become what is in reality the unfulfilled dream of a parent. Or — and here's where it gets tricky — wanting to succeed but adhering to an unconscious agreement not to surpass the success of a parent lest he or she be envious and not love us. Abraham Maslow writes about the compassionate sacrifice, that is, to make yourself wrong or less in order to protect the illusion. We will all too often sacrifice our dreams in order to be loved or accepted. And even when we do, it seldom works.

Yes, we are complex beings. So it is vital to know ourselves and the undercurrents of our psyche as well as possible. This way we will be living our lives as who we truly are, unencumbered by illusions.

Let us explore other possible undercurrents of desire.

In a creative act of desire, sometimes imagined images take on lives of their own.

Psyche or our unconscious can dictate a greater allure than the real thing. Hence, even after achieving a strong desire, we may remain unsatisfied or disappointed with the reality of the desired object. This is because what is imagined and idealized can be much more than the actual object of desire. Remember my desired red shoes? Dorothy's were magical shoes given by Glinda, the Good Witch. The ones I purchased in New York were not.

So an ardent desire process must work itself through. This is how the lessons are learned. This is how we may one day grow beyond the desire nature. So by buying those red shoes after wanting them for so many years, I did myself a great service. I experienced that fulfilling my desire only bought temporary — not permanent — happiness. The moment the object of my fulfilled desire ceased to make me happy, I learned a valuable lesson. So, for that, I am eternally grateful.

EXERCISE

Think of something you wanted very much when you were young, but which you did not get. Years later, you bought or achieved it for yourself. Describe how the wanting felt, what it was you craved, and how it felt later on when it was yours. How long did that feeling last?

Wanting What Is Past

No man is rich enough to buy back his past.
   Oscar Wilde

Art Buchwald was right when he spoke of how we seem to be going through a time of nostalgia, believing that yesterday was better than today. Was it really? Madison Avenue makes billions by marketing our nostalgia for the past. Is there anyone who really would like to go back to high school again? Of course, it is fun or at least interesting to look back and remember. That's all right, but just don't get stuck where what was is no more. The past is a good place to visit, but I wouldn't want to live there.

In the last chapter, we explored the concept of dharma or the inner law of your existence. Sometimes we identify with what served as dharma yesterday and cease to notice when it may change. Nonetheless, another amazing thing about following dharma is that when you are fully committed to your inner calling, even unknowingly you will slip into the right place or meet the right person at the right time. Or be a magnet for what is needed to fulfill your dharma. It seems to be a law unto itself. Who hasn't run into someone you know yet haven't seen for ages, and later on discover that there was a hidden reason for you to come together? Or who hasn't picked up a magazine or book that carries vital information for what you need to know now? This is psyche at work. And this will intensify when centered and in touch with dharma.

Sometimes what we want to be is not what our dharma is. Hopefully, sooner or later, awareness will manifest to discover what it is we are truly meant to do. *Mr. Holland's Opus* is a wonderful movie, based on a true story, starring Richard Dreyfuss. It's the story of a man who dreamed of being a composer and, in order to survive, takes a job teaching music in a high school. He discovers in time that his true calling was to be a great teacher instead.

Here's another example. As a young man in Denmark, Hans Christian Andersen (1805–75) went to a psychic who told him that one day he would become famous, and when he returned home, people would be lined up in the streets to cheer him. Well, Andersen's dream was to become an opera singer so he assumed that this meant he would become a famous singer. He wrote fairy tales yet didn't think they were anything special. And, of course, it is the amazing fairy tales — over one hundred and fifty — that the Danish author is famous for. Indeed, as the psychic predicted, when Hans Christian Andersen returned to his island home, people lined the streets to cheer him!

It is indeed better to follow dharma than to be something fate did not intend. Sometimes the individual may not be aware so fate has to step in and nudge. Here's another literary example.

Louisa May Alcott (1832–88) was a moderately successful commercial writer of gothic novels. Her publisher had been asking her for some time to write a book for children, especially young female readers. Totally uninterested, she declined again and again, identifying herself as a writer of gothic novels. That is, until the wily publisher offered to publish her philosopher-father's writings if she would write one book for young girls. So, drawing from her own life and family, as well as her three sisters, she wrote a novel called *Little Women*, and the rest is history. The book was a sensation and from then on, Alcott wrote only for young readers. Dharma was working despite her initial resistance. And helpers — both physical and subtle — arose to show the way.

EXERCISE

Think of an unexpected incident or situation that became a turning point in your life, one which somehow served your dharma calling. Write about it.

The Many Names of Wealth

When asked, "What thing about humanity surprises you the most?" Tibet's Dalai Lama once answered:

Man.... Because he sacrifices his health in order to make money. Then he sacrifices money to recuperate his health. And then he is so anxious about the future that he does not enjoy the present; the result being that he does not live in the present or the future; he lives as if he is never going to die, and then dies having never really lived.

Years ago when I was a young actor in New York, I went to an opening night party of a play I was performing in, and met a doctor in his mid-thirties. He admitted to being envious of my life in the theatre and confessed to me that he had always wanted to be an actor himself. "Then why don't you?" I asked. "Well, you see, my father was a doctor and had his heart set on my being one. Then I married and now have children to support. So I'm a doctor, and a very successful one at that." I never saw the man again but always remembered the unmistakable look of regret on his face that night. He was earning many times the amount I was at that time, yet somehow I felt far richer.

> *Don't play for safety. It's the most dangerous thing in the world.*
> Hugh Walpole

People, like the doctor, have a hundred reasons for not living their dreams and a hundred forms of fear. Mostly it is a fear of not earning enough money to survive, take care of their families, or live as comfortably as they wish. It is challenging today to think of survival in any other terms except a monetary one. Times are uncertain economically. Many who settled for security and gave decades to large corporations are suddenly let go, wondering why they gave up their dream for this. Yes, times are uncertain these days, but one thing has always been constant, if we are aware. An inner truth exists in each of us, regardless of outer forces. Outer circumstances fluctuate all the time, inner truth never.

> *Happiness is when what you say, what you do and what you think is in harmony.*
> Mohandas Gandhi

Mohandas Gandhi was a young lawyer with a promising career ahead, and yet he gave his life to one ideal: the pursuit of truth. This manifested as a mission for the independence of India. This was his dharma, and though certainly challenging, resulted in fulfillment.

> *Follow your bliss. There's something inside you that knows when you're in the center, that knows when you're on the beam or off the beam. And if you get off the beam to earn money, you've lost your life. And if you stay in the center and don't get any money, you still have your bliss.*
> Joseph Campbell

Wealth is defined in *Webster's II New Riverside University Dictionary* as "abundance of valuable material possessions or resources." However there are two other definitions that follow this one: "the state of being rich" and "a profusion of abundance."

How many times have you stood before a glorious sunset with someone you loved and felt a profusion of abundance? How often have you enjoyed the presence of good friends or family over a delicious meal and experienced the richness of life?

I recently went with my seven-year-old grandson to feed the ducks at a nearby lake. It was his first time to feed the ducks and he was as excited as I've ever seen anyone be excited. In this shared experience, I felt a profusion of abundance. And the experience was absolutely free!

EXERCISE

Remember a moment of abundance in your life. First describe a time you felt a state of being rich and then describe a moment that gave you a profusion of abundance.

Conversely, how often have you known someone with great material wealth who was not happy, perhaps not even healthy, and maybe had difficulty trusting others for fear they liked him or her only because of the wealth? Or the fear that others were there to get something from them?

Many years ago, on my first schoolgirl summer in Europe, I was in Capri, Italy — one of the loveliest places in the world. There I met a woman in her mid-thirties who invited me to join her for lunch. She confided that she was the heiress of a vast American industrial fortune (which shall remain nameless). Later, a handsome young Italian couple joined us at the table. After introducing us, she sent them away saying she would shortly join them. After they left, she explained that she had hired them to make love, and asked me if I would care to join her to watch! Only nineteen, I was at first shocked and then saddened that with all this inherited wealth, this is how she chose to use it. I declined her invitation, and instead took a solitary walk along the cliff overlooking the Mediterranean, allowing the wind to cleanse.

The first important question is what is wealth to you? For a happy life, it is terribly important to differentiate your individual values from those of the world. Words might arise such as family, friends, health, meaningful work, some life purpose, perhaps a spiritual life.

EXERCISE

Consider how you would define wealth — not in the world's view — but in yours. Write down your definition. Then make a list of what you would require in your life in order to feel true abundance.

Past Regrets

Finish each day and be done with it.
You have done what you could; some blunders
and absurdities have crept in; forget them
as soon as you can. Tomorrow is a new day;
you shall begin it serenely and with too high a
spirit to be encumbered with your old nonsense.
Ralph Waldo Emerson

Do you feel you have to achieve in order to receive acceptance or love? Did you get the message while young, "I am not worthy. Only what I do matters, not who I am."

When love is not there, as a child, we feel something is wrong with us. We feel it is not enough to be loved for ourselves alone. We must do something to earn that love. How to re-nurture ourselves? Initially the feeling of grief and rage may arise as we slowly become aware of what wasn't there for us when young. Allow yourself to feel it then let it go.

Tomorrow Is Another Day

If you wait for tomorrow, tomorrow comes.
If you don't wait for tomorrow, tomorrow comes.
Senegalese saying

As with Scarlett O'Hara, when in the grip of an uncontrollable desire, projecting that tomorrow might succeed helps us get through the night. However, if we are not facing and being in the now, tomorrow may be lost, as well.

Spend sufficient time discovering who you are and what you are meant to do.

Live from that knowing center in yourself, and it will guide you, pointing the way to what you are to do now. Be prepared though to make changes, if necessary.

When you want something you've never had, you may have to do something you've never done.

Whom We Love and Why

The friend or lover who rejects me is the one I will yearn for, call, and think about. Sound like anyone you know? I can track this tendency in myself to my own history. My father left the family when I was four. When there are abandonment issues, there may be an obsessive-compulsive behavior toward people who are distant or who leave. Though not logical, it is deeply felt. Though it may never entirely leave us, we can cultivate ways of stepping back and, with compassion, witness these tendencies in ourselves. Understanding ourselves is a powerful tool to change our actions. Patterns are set in motion when we are young, and it sometimes takes years of inner work to sort them out. Once sorted, however, they have less negative power in our lives. (Of course, good patterns are also imprinted, as well.)

What We Love and Why

I can remember as a child after a trip to the dentist or getting straight A's in school being rewarded by chocolate. Even now, I reward myself with chocolate — now, dark chocolate. The little child within us lives on long past puberty and even adulthood.

(I am grateful to modern science, which declares that dark chocolate is good for us!)

Of course, many early childhood imprints are quite positive, installing positive patterns of what we love years and years later. For instance, swimming — especially in rivers, lakes, or oceans — became for me a lasting joy.

Also, as an only child, I learned early to be alone and take refuge in solitude. Often the happiest times were spent lying on the grass and gazing at slow-moving clouds above. Time stopped and I was in myself. I still love to cloud-gaze and recognize it now as a kind of meditation. It stills my monkey mind and centers me in a way unlike anything else. Nature is a great friend — if we open to her.

EXERCISE

Think of two imprints from childhood that have created a continuing pattern of what you love. Write down the origin and also how it manifests in your life today.

The Continuous Thread of Revelation

*Events in our lives happen in a sequence
of time, but in their significance to ourselves,
they find their own order... the continuous
thread of revelation.*
Eudora Welty

Have you ever found yourself blocked from doing what you've done well for years, even decades? At these times, you may often become confused — even mystified.

As we grow, we develop certain skills after much focus and effort. We get used to doing what we do well and what works, which sometimes leads to a reluctance to expand or try something new. Habit takes over, and we may not even be aware that on some level we are blocked from expanding our limits. When something works, why explore elsewhere? Of course, sooner or later we learn that something only works until it doesn't work.

Here's an example from my own life. I had worked for years writing plays in New York then writing film and television in Hollywood. My field was dramatic writing. I knew who I was and was identified with what I had always done. For some reason, I stopped writing, had a long writer's block, and became depressed. How could I think of myself as a writer when I could not write? After completing two assignments in Hollywood, I felt emptied out and needed to replenish my well. So I took a break and visited friends in Santa Fe. There I became a total slug, lying in a hammock, watching clouds pass overhead. (The clouds and sky in New Mexico are rather

35

terrific!) I finally stopped resisting and let go of everything, allowing myself to drift and dream. I even let go of expectation. In this woozy state, I heard a small, clear voice within say, "The Way of Story." Then an epiphany came and I knew I was to write a book whose title was *The Way of Story*. You see, I had never before written a book, and so I kept trying to write what I had written for decades, i.e., plays and screenplays. I thanked my friends, returned home to California, stopped trying to find work in Hollywood, and took time out to research and write my first book, a nonfiction, partial memoir book on writing, *The Way of Story: The Craft and Soul of Writing*. It was this book that became a turning point in my own dharma — both teaching and writing.

So the point is sometimes a block may simply mean *what you've always done no longer serves*. It is no longer the road to take. Similarly, sometimes depression arises to send a message that the patterns which have become habitual need to be changed. They just don't work anymore. This means we have to change the story of who we are and what we are about. This might mean spiritual changes, leaving a marriage, moving to another town, or choosing another career. Again, courage is needed for these transitions, as it may demand from us a leap into the unknown. The unknown can, in fact, be a very creative place to be.

The bottom line is we are here to grow, and without change, there is no growth.

So it is perhaps important to be open to change and to keep your radar tuned for inner voices and outer signs to help point the way.

The adventure of life is to learn.
The goal of life is to grow.
The nature of life is to change.
The challenge of life is to overcome.
The essence of life is to care.
The secret of life is to dare.
The beauty of life is to give.
The joy of life is to love.
William Arthur Ward

EXERCISE

Think of a time in your life where you were blocked and couldn't move forward, yet later realized it was because you needed to change something in your life — people, place, work, behavior, whatever. Write the before, what gave you the epiphany, and what the new life was. And express your gratitude for taking the road not travelled.

How to Want What We Have?

At around age seven, I heard a record of the book and Disney film *So Dear to My Heart*. It is the story of a young boy who lives in the rural South with his grandmother, and is very, very poor. The boy dreams of raising a champion racehorse and winning a blue ribbon at the county fair. Instead of a horse, he only gets a black lamb. One rainy evening, he opens a book and an animated owl jumps out and sings, "You got to do with what you got." So even though a black sheep had never won a ribbon before, he raises that lamb and takes him to the county fair. It surprises everyone when Jeremiah Kincaid wins a special blue ribbon for his black sheep. Somehow this story and simple lesson imprinted itself on my seven-year-old mind. Even today, I try and "Do with what I got" and not waste my life dreaming of what I don't have. Thank you, Walt Disney!

EXERCISE

Think of something you have that may have potential if only you do something with it. It can be a talent, an idea, a friendship, a place, a dream — whatever is there now. Write about it. What are the possibilities? What do you need in order to make something from what you've got? You have to first know what you need in order to ask for it.

The funny thing is that quite often what I want is not the best thing in the long run while what is already there or comes of its own — often unexpectedly — is better than anything I had wished for! So perhaps what is required is a lessening of desires and instead an opening to what is best for the soul's journey. Remain vigilant with a silent mind, and trust that the universe will provide the very best for your individual journey.

Nothing is worth more than this day.
Johann Wolfgang von Goethe

Chapter Three

Balancing Thinking
with Feeling

---

*Feeling and longing are the motive forces
behind all human endeavor and human
creations.*
  Albert Einstein

Why when we have so much do we feel so insecure? Why do our feelings leave us wanting when materially we have more than most? Perhaps it is because, in part, we think too much and feel too little. Why is this? Perhaps one cause is that both at home and in school, we are conditioned to think and not to feel. From a very young age, we are trained to think and to value what we think. In most schools, budgets for right brain activities are the first to be cut. Value is not given equally to what we feel. In most schools, right-brain activities are cut first. To excel in math or science matters while the arts, which help develop feelings, do not.

How often today have our young people spoken of being lost, not being one's self, or being split off from themselves? How many victims of trauma have spoken of feeling disconnected from the body at the moment of trauma — and even years afterwards?

Feeling carries a special power in the lives of young people. Far better to allow youth a safe container for their dark side rather than to have them self-destruct or commit a crime. Today we are shocked and mystified by the increase in random homicides of innocent strangers. One solution may be to offer a safe and appropriate outlet for the confusion and despair happening within so many of us today. To harbor dark feelings is not a crime. To harbor dark feelings is a natural part of being human. Creativity offers a suitable outlet for these dark feelings.

I witnessed a transforming effect over and over again when I was asked by the Dramatists Guild to help launch the Young Playwrights Program in the New York City public schools. I joined Tony Award-winning playwright Terrence McNally and others and ventured out into junior high and high schools all over New York, teaching playwriting workshops in a range of neighborhoods as diverse as the Upper East Side of Manhattan to Harlem and the South Bronx. After several classes using improvisations to teach dramatic writing, we would encourage the students to write a one-act play then enter it into the annual national competition, the Young Playwrights Festival. The winners, ages eight to nineteen, would have a professional off-Broadway production in New York and afterwards, Avon Books would publish their plays. This ambitious project gave value to creative writing and to those who wrote, and the results were absolutely amazing! Full productions were mounted at Joseph Papp's Public Theatre and at Playwrights Horizons, enabling the young writers to see their plays come alive with professional actors. One writer was all of eight years old!

*Theatre glamorizes thought and reveals the
human heart. This makes it as important
as the scientist, psychologist, or minister.*
  Laurence Olivier

How to convince government today that cultivating
the arts is essential to a balanced society? Creativity and
putting value on what we feel is not simply for artists. Regardless of whether one becomes a professional creative
or not is beside the point. The arts are necessary in order
to develop the heart and elevate one's feelings. And, without heart, we are in danger. "The world hangs on a slender
thread," Jung wrote, "and that is the psyche of man."

*Art establishes the basic human truths which
must serve as the touchstones of our judgment.
The artist, however faithful to his vision of
reality, becomes the last champion of the
individual mind and sensibility against an
intrusive society.*
  John F. Kennedy

What world do you wish to live in today? What are
the models you will offer to your children? What world
will you create?

The way we think creates our feelings. And the way
we feel dictates how we think. From this comes the
driving force of desire, what we want, what we long for.

So best to be aware of what you long for.

EXERCISE

———

Make a list of what you long for. What is it you value and want more than anything else?

Now make a list of what you long to do to change your world for the better.

> *I have made my world and it is a much*
> *better world than I ever saw outside.*
> Louise Nevelson, sculptor

Ultimately, we long for what we truly are. In fact, we long for what is our essence. And we don't long from our left logical brain, but from some deeper place within, from a deeper, *feeling* Self.

All of life is a capacity for presence, to be fully in the moment, to be present. The greatest gift to another is presence. What if you were able to truly listen to a loved one, to offer him or her the gift of your presence?

EXERCISE

———

Think back to a moment when someone was there for you, someone who was truly present during a difficult or transitional moment in your life. Write about it. What did you feel? Now remember a time you were present for someone. Write about that. What did you feel then?

To be fully present requires true listening. Listening is more than simply recalling what you know. Listening is an art. Listening without judgment is love. Why is listening without judgment such a challenge? What gets in the way?

Usually, when we have had a critical parent, we grow up to judge others in a similar fashion. It is possible to become aware of what you are thinking or feeling as distinct from what your inner parent is thinking or feeling. The more you develop this awareness, the less you will feel the need or impulse to express such a judgmental thought or feeling upon others or even yourself.

Though imprinted early on, the internalized parent resides in our unconscious. As a mother, I have had moments when my son was young, when I caught myself reacting exactly how my mother would. Then the moment came when I thought, "That's not me. That's my mother." The negative judgmental thought would lessen and I would feel more myself again and more present for my son. Later on when such a thought arose, I would simply say to myself, with gentle humor, "Thank you, Mother, but no thank you."

EXERCISE

Think of a time when you reacted not as yourself but as an internalized parent. What was the result? Write it down.

Thinking Has Its Place

Of course, thinking does have its place, but best not to allow it to occupy all of you. Let the mind serve something higher, something deeper. Let it be a servant — not a dictator. Jung commented once that the mind is the servant of the soul. The problem is that too many are following the servant.

Once we know who we are in the deepest sense, the mind can serve our dharma and inner path. It can become a guard so that we do not go astray from our chosen path or soul essence. It can offer discrimination of what is right and wrong, not only from an ethical and moral view, but from a spiritual perspective, as well. For instance, through experience, discrimination can inform us of which thoughts and action bring us closer to enlightenment and which take us further from a spiritual goal. In fact, the mind can be a powerful ally as long as it is not given full sway over how you live your life. Make room for the heart's voice and intuition as well. (More on intuition will follow in the next chapter.) Your heart will tell you the right direction. Once this is known, the mind can help organize and manifest that right direction. How to discover that right direction? Feel it. Ask yourself what makes me happy in the deepest sense? What gives me a sense of fulfillment? Then do more of that. Remember that something deep within always knows. We have only to listen with our heart. And listen well.

A great French mathematician and writer once presented a method to find any solution:

All of man's problems come from his inability to sit quietly in a room alone.
Blaise Pascal

How often when we are faced with a problem do we look for distraction, our monkey minds going in every direction, away from stillness, away from Self. Disconnected thinking destroys life and rarely delivers true and lasting answers. Sometimes all that is needed is to stop monkeying around and simply sit quietly, embrace stillness, and listen to that still inner voice within.

Sometimes it is helpful to use forms of oracles such as astrology, cards, or the *I Ching* as a way to focus on the problem in such a manner as to allow the intuitive to aid us. These can be an invitation to what I call "the invisibles" — allies who come to our aid. The intention behind using forms of oracle is perhaps the most important aspect of this process and not the device or tool itself.

Automatic writing can also be a form of meditation and centering. Sometimes it is useful to spend some time with closed eyes, pleasant music, and incense or candle before the act of automatic writing. Centering, inviting subtle guides, or simply finding a deeper part of ourselves all serve as potential tools for self-discovery. Just meditate on the problem and then start writing without thinking. Write without knowing what you are writing about. (In the next chapter, "Soul Dialogues: Getting In Touch with the Inner Visionary," you will find more exercises to serve as a jumpstart.)

Whichever method you adopt, the amazing thing is that when you still the mind, listen deeply from the heart, the way will present itself — in time. It may take a spot of time but the answer is there, and will come, if you are patient. It is best to remember that the answer comes not always in your own time, but in *its* own time.

EXERCISE

Breathe deeply, focusing on the area between the heart and solar plexus. Close your eyes and breathe from the soul, ask for the guidance needed. Be still and feel whatever comes, then write it down.

As Jung has stated, the collective unconscious is always there ready to heal us. We need only become conscious of our personal unconscious. This constitutes the necessary inner work that leads to healing and becoming whole. Healing is only another word for becoming whole.

Another blessing is that when we deeply attend to the inner work of discerning our voice from the internalized voices of others within us, there is no need to forgive wrongs done to us in the past. No forgiveness is required when we let go of the past, and are fully present in ourselves.

Heaven or Hell, love or hate
No matter where I turn
I meet myself.
Holding life is precious is
Just living with all intensity
Holding life precious.
   Kosho Uchiyama Roshi

Opening to Allow Feeling

There is a story of the Chinese Zen teacher, Hogen, who lived alone in a small temple in the country. One day four travelling monks came and asked if they could make a fire in his yard to keep warm. As they were building the fire, Hogen overheard them arguing about philosophy. He asked them, "See that big stone over there?" They replied, "Yes." Then the Teacher said, "Is it inside or outside your mind?" When one of the monks replied, "It is inside my mind," Hogen said, "Your head must feel very heavy if you are carrying around a stone like that in your mind." After this, the monks experienced no more argument, only a silent mind.

Sometimes a period of unlearning is needed in order to allow deeper feelings to arise. How many times have I heard artists or musicians or writers say that after their training, they had to *unlearn* in order to be free enough to create. It is not only creatives who say this. Once a lawyer told me there was such a gap between law school and real-life practice that he had to spend time "unlearning" before he could practice law well. Nothing closes our mind to learning more than thinking we already know. Remember the cup must be empty in order to receive. The big stone must be removed from our minds. When we act only from studied learning, there is no space for the feeling or intuitive part of us to act. And sometimes this "space" is just what is needed.

Also, the mad pace of life today all too often prevents the necessary stillness for us to listen to deeper parts of ourselves. The very speed of life today influences us to live more on the surface of ourselves, sometimes re-pressing who we truly are. This is why I try almost each year to return to India — my spiritual home — for a personal retreat. When friends ask me what I do there, I say, "Absolutely nothing." It is essential to program time to do nothing. There is a need for time to simply be still, time to check in with the rest of what constitutes the Self. From there, all else comes.

> *Therefore the sage goes about doing nothing,*
> *teaching no-talking.*
> *The ten thousand things rise and fall without*
> *cease, Creating, yet not.*
> *Working, yet not taking credit.*
> *Work is done then forgotten.*
> *Therefore it lasts forever.*
>   Lao Tzu, *Tao te King*

When It Hurts to Feel

There is a part of us that just doesn't want to feel be-cause to feel is to react rather than respond, to remember past wounds from life and/or from others. So we systematically set about ways not to feel. Alcohol. Drugs. Overeating. Sex. Television. Work. Perhaps flu flares and we are forced to be still. Often this comes as a relief. To just drop out of life for a while and allow ourselves to let go and drift. So what we avoid — being still — is forced upon us and a kind of surrender is required. This surrender itself can take us not only to healing, but a step toward integration and wholeness. Without judgment, hold the awareness that there may always be a part of us that just doesn't want to be fully here. Though part of us wants to be whole and present, another part pulls away from being present and works against our greater good. Sometimes the universe sends us "stoppers" such as an unexpected illness or accident which may become an ally on our journey, causing us to stop and be still.

To avoid this, it is better to take the time before such events arise. The truth is that dropping out for a time is healthy — especially if we do it consciously. Meditation is one way. Sit for ten or twenty minutes each morning and choose whatever meditation or discipline appeals. Best do it in the same place each time, if possible. This builds up an atmosphere that adds more ease in each sitting to go deeper. Some people get the same effect by spending time in their garden — especially when alone.

Years ago, I was living in an ashram in India, and the Sage was suggesting the benefits of daily meditation. An older woman from France was there and in her outspoken manner, quipped, "I never meditate." Now this woman had been following the spiritual path for many years and was very sincere. The Sage gently asked her what she did when she got up in the morning. "Well, I have a cup of coffee. Then I go out into my garden, look at my roses, and think of the Sage." The Sage smiled and said, "That is meditation."

There is no one path to truth. Meditation is not only sitting in a corner with closed eyes. Your *vasanas* or inborn tendencies will point the way. Just follow the one that appeals, and go to the end of it. If the path you choose seems lacking and if you are earnest, something or someone will appear to light the way to a more suitable path. Something within naively, intuitively urges us in the direction of our destined unfolding. Even when circumstances seem unfavorable at a given time, the process is at work. Who has not experienced being stuck in a meaningless job or relationship or circumstance, yet that very situation in time opens a pathway to our true destiny.

This reminds me of the old story about the farmer and his son. First their stallion runs away and is missing for three days. The farmer bemoans his bad luck, that is, until the stallion returns with a mare. Now with two horses instead of one, all is well, that is, until his son, only eighteen, falls off the horse and breaks his leg. The farmer bemoans their bad luck, that is, until the army comes around enlisting all the young men. They cannot take a young boy with a broken leg so he is left to stay at home and help his father. Who can know when seeming bad fortune is really good fortune in the long run.

Or when even a negative event in our lives can be just what is needed for the growth of the soul.

Daily attention to inner life can provide the courage to face the challenging feelings and events that inevitably arise in a life lived. With this ballast, you can sail through such feelings without suppressing them. The amazing thing is that when we allow feelings without resistance, step back, and simply become aware of them, they often eventually transform themselves!

Man is the only animal that is both social and solitary. Some may require more of one than the other, but the plain fact is that both are needed for a balanced life. To be with others may sometimes result in a greater loneliness. To be alone need not be lonely.

EXERCISE

Read the following poem by Wordsworth and read it slowly. Allow space between the words and see what arises from within. Read it twice if needed then write whatever associations come.

> *When from our better selves we have too long*
> *Been parted by the hurrying world, and droop,*
> *Sick of its business, of its pleasures tired,*
> *How gracious, how benign is Solitude.*
> *For oft, when on my couch I lie*
> *In vacant or in pensive mood,*
> *They flash upon that inward eye*
> *Which is the bliss of solitude;*
> *And then my heart with pleasure fills*
> *And dances with the daffodils.*
>   William Wordsworth

A Return to Innocence

When a kind of transformation occurs, you may experience a feeling of a return to innocence. Yet this requires setting aside time needed to descend to the depths of feeling, time to commune with the roses, the daffodils, and oneself. Therein lies treasure and a return to innocence.

EXERCISE

What activity, book, film, music, or nature experience helps you return to a feeling of innocence? Write about it.

Feelings Beyond One's Self

In ancient times, around a campfire, the tribe would gather to listen to a story of some climatic event. It may have been a hunter relating how his friend or father or brother had been killed by an animal or a neighboring tribesman. Expressing and listening to one's story is an ancient mode of healing. Responding to another's suffering with compassion is an essential part of being human.

The very word compassion means "shared sorrow." For sorrow to become compassion, it must be shared or expressed to others. Sometimes expanding our specific sorrow or wound to embrace all others who have suffered a similar wrong or injury can alleviate our own.

There has been an avalanche of memoir in recent years. A large percentage of contemporary memoirs published today deal with experiencing and recovering from a life trauma, such as serious physical or psychological illness, accident, war trauma, or abuse of some kind. Each day, thirteen American war veterans commit suicide. Writing a memoir is often an attempt at self-healing — consciously or unconsciously. And yet, the dimension that I feel often missing in modern true stories is a wider arc of compassion touching all those who have suffered. As a result, these books may sometimes even border on self-indulgence. Often we feel as if no one has suffered what we have suffered and that no one else can understand the suffering we have gone through, and yet, suffering is as universal as love. Actually, to suffer offers us the opportunity to understand the suffering of others. It only requires of us one more small step.

Sometimes when overwhelmed with life's challenges, we isolate ourselves. This last exercise is a step toward expanding beyond ourselves. While we need solitude, we also need the company of others. Foster in yourself the courage to be fully present in whatever state you find yourself. Be true to what you are feeling.

> *Whatever you do, you should do it*
> *with feeling.*
> Yogi Berra

EXERCISE

Close your eyes and let arise in your mind a specific sorrow or suffering you have experienced. Hold the vision of this for a moment. Breathe into it. Now envision a white light as you inhale and draw into your body this sorrow. Let it fill your body. Envision whatever color or image it may take. Be still and allow this feeling. Now visualize your individual suffering expanding, encircling all souls who have suffered as you have. Experience this white shining light expanding. Experience how your own suffering is now transformed into the bright white light of compassion for all. Breathe easily in and out, transmuting the energy of pain and sorrow into that of love and compassion for all who have suffered in this world.

In order to balance thinking and feeling, it is necessary to feel and not repress what we are feeling. Becoming more aware of what you are feeling will help to clarify your thinking as well. Clarity arises from balance. To achieve balance, it is better to open our eyes and gaze beyond ourselves.

Life is a face of truth, mirroring back to us, ourselves.

Chapter Four

Soul Dialogues: Getting In Touch with the Inner Visionary

Stay at your table and listen. Don't even listen, just wait, be completely quiet and alone. The world will offer itself to you to be unmasked.
Franz Kafka

Accessing and communicating with the inner visionary is the best method for self-healing as well as expanding your world both within and without. A famous mathematician from India called Ramanujan, who later studied at Cambridge University, was asked how he came up with such remarkable mathematical discoveries while he was only a humble clerk from Madras. He replied that at night when he was asleep, Devi (goddess) would come and whisper in his ear, telling him the solutions.

As soon as the least of us stands still that's the moment something extraordinary is seen to be going on in the world.
Eudora Welty

A human being sometimes needs to do nothing. He may seem to be doing nothing yet in fact he is tuning out of the outer world in order to allow the inner intuitive mind to drift and dream. For those who remember, before television and computer games, there was cloud-gazing — a spiritual, introspective pursuit with no goal whatsoever.

> *I saw myself when I shut my eyes: space,*
> *space, where I am and am not.*
>   Octavio Paz, Nobel Prize-winning poet

When my son was three, we lived in a small village in south India. What toys he had were made from banana palm, coconut palm leaf, and other natural substances. However, I did manage to obtain paper and crayons from a nearby town. One morning, I asked him to draw "love" and without hesitation he drew two wide blue circles. Young children do not have a sense of the right or wrong way to draw anything. They do not hesitate to draw a purple sky or red grass. They are not afraid to draw outside the lines. They create empty spaces to play.

Of course, this is so only of the very young preschool child, for quite soon this wonderfully imaginative child will be conditioned away from freely inhabiting this empty space. He will be *educated* into right and wrong, good and bad, and all manner of comparatives that inhibit the pure spontaneity of creating space. He will become conscious of the right way to do things. "The sky must be blue; the grass only green." Thus creation becomes less and less necessary — even extinct.

This chapter is about creating a space for your soul to play. It's about letting go and letting your creativity arise like a dream from your unconscious. In a way, it's about learning to be three again.

To write is to create a space in which things
can happen. To live one's life, the same.
Michael Adam, *Man is a Little World*

Remember, a culture defines itself by what it values. Once I heard an interview with Joseph Campbell and Bill Moyers. Campbell was saying how what we value at different times in history is illustrated by what is built in the center of town. For instance, during the Middle Ages, the church or cathedral was the center of the society. During the Renaissance, the buildings to house the government or whoever ruled became the center. Now it is the mercantile buildings of corporations that are the center of our lives. Who we become is in response to what is valued or made central to our lives. Targeting the World Trade Towers on September 11, 2001, was a calculated choice to hit at the center of America.

Beware the effects of a fragmented society. Perhaps someone should express concern about having to live in a society where creativity is not only undervalued, but all but ignored. Creativity is vital for a balanced society, that is, in the schools, not because one might become an artist one day, but because the arts develop the heart — not only the rational mind. I don't know about anyone else, but I would hope that whoever holds the power to push the red button for nuclear war had a balanced education of both heart and mind. I would hope my President had read Shakespeare, listened to Mozart, and, in a moment of stillness, pondered Monet's paintings of the Givenchy water lilies.

Like dreams, creativity arises from the unconscious. We have to create an empty space in our conscious minds for the unconscious to emerge with its gifts. Our conditioning prods us to rush in with interpretative meaning, learned meanings, which may only serve to flatten the true value of what arises naturally from within. Mental understanding won't necessarily change us. To be transformed requires something more than rational thinking or sentimentalism. The conditioned way of mental knowing often strengthens the ego at the expense of soul. In fact, mere mental understanding may be overrated today. Logical thinking — though a valuable tool — is only handmaiden to a far deeper process.

Real doing comes from stillness — not endless busyness or even reading. Perhaps now is a good time to stop and do the following exercise.

EXERCISE

Sit quietly for a moment and simply feel your body. Now imagine you are naked lying in the sun. Stay with the feeling, feel it specifically all over your body. Now allow your mind to free associate. You might think of someone you love or when you were a small child. Go with the images. Now pick up your pen and write about some past peak experience where the feelings are raw and visceral.

Body Dialogue

During my training in Depth Psychology, I read a small but important book called *Focusing* by Eugene T. Gendlin. It guides the reader to include the body in our response to life and to our dreams. There is now a new field called *somatic psychology*. For too long, spirit was emphasized with the exclusion of the body. This was especially true in organized monotheistic religions. A life of spirit is not enough. One requires soul. And soul includes mind, spirit, and body. It is important never to forget this.

As with many type-A personalities, relaxation wasn't all that natural for me. We all have one part of the body that when tense, suffers. With me, it is the neck. Sometimes these knots of tension in my neck can be quite painful. I used to massage the knot, trying to release the tension, yet the knot persisted. Then I started asking the knot what it wanted me to know, what I needed to learn. Once I began to do this, the knots, having been "heard," often dissipate.

EXERCISE

Sit quietly with closed eyes. Feel which part of your body is struggling or tense. Then after taking and releasing a breath, talk to it. Ask this part of you what it wishes you to know, what you need to learn. Listen then write it down. After doing so, thank this part of your body for communicating in this way.

Awakening the Inner Eye

All things create themselves from their own innermost reflection and none can tell how they came to do so.
   Chang Tzu

Even before there are thoughts, there are images. Each life is formed by its unique image, an image that is the essence of that life and that calls it to destiny. To discover the image, we must enter the invisible world and allow it to carry us. Intuitive images occur; we cannot make them. All we can do is get out of the way, thereby inviting them to come through.

Images are the natural language of the unconscious. Psyche is revealed through images as in dreams. Sometimes the darkest image may prove the most valuable. Consider Kafka's cockroach in *Metamorphosis* or Dante's images of hell in his *Inferno*. So don't censor what images emerge. Simply remain centered in yourself and watch them with awareness.

The intolerable image is the transformational image.
   Wallace Stevens

Images are the language of the soul. They integrate mind, body, and soul and thereby serve a healing function. The metaphorical or symbolic image lifts the reader from the gross level to a realm of poetry where image and soul reign. This is where transformation occurs.

EXERCISE

Take a moment, visualize standing in an open field, looking upward at a clear blue sky. Now sink deep into yourself before writing. Close your eyes, feel what is going on within. Then without undue thought, pick up your pen and write whatever wants to come. On channeling: Let it come through you, not from you. Dare to be surprised!

Some version of the above exercise might become a simple, daily ritual. You might light a candle or do a brief meditation or simply take and release deep breaths inviting whatever images might knock on your door. Or you can play music that makes you soar. In this way, a dimension of the sacred is added as well as an invitation extended to invisible helpers or guides.

If you think of it, the moments remembered in a great novel or film are usually visual moments, unspoken moments. Virtual reality without technology. Memory is one of the primal sources for creative images. We may find ourselves experiencing reality on more than one plane. The creative act is thus an act of liberation — the defeat of habit by originality. The creative process does not travel in straight lines. It thrives in the undefined spaces in between.

EXERCISE

Visualize a family photo of one of your parents, grandparents, or a lover. Sit quietly in front of the photograph, allowing your mind to drift into memories of things past. Close your eyes. Try to remember how this person smelled. Recall his or her touch. Then, whether the experience is positive or negative, describe it in words from a *feeling* perspective. Find an image (bird, animal, or object) to represent this person and how he or she would move and behave.

Jungian analyst James Hillman said the aim of the dream is to redress a supposed lost balance. As a conditioned child who had lost her empty space, I had been educated away from a deeper soul balance. A series of owl dreams came to redress this balance, to center me. But the experience came not from mental activity, but by letting go of the gathering busy mind, sinking down into the body, and allowing the dream image to work itself on me. In other words, the owl image had moved from concept to experience. Experience — though spiritual in nature — is grounded in body awareness. As a child filling empty space, I had invited the dream image of the owl to inhabit me. And it was good.

You might keep your journal next to your bedside and when awakening from a dream, write it down. Dreams are the way that our unconscious communicates to us. Let intuition guide you through metaphor or symbolic images. Create a habit of listening inwardly. Before sleep, ask for a dream. It is through metaphor that the process of life and art can be seen as in a mirror. Look for metaphors in both waking and dream states. Awaken that part of the mind that generates images. Dare to explore the unknown regions of the psyche, for therein lie alchemical gold.

Here's a visualization exercise that can begin to tap hidden resources. And never forget that the most valuable resource is your own Self. Approach the blank page as if for the first time. You might choose to play some sacred or soothing music. This exercise serves as an invocation and ritual to summon the Muse or Inner Guide. (If possible, ask a friend to read it out loud to you so you can close your eyes and give yourself over to this inner journey.)

EXERCISE

Close your eyes. Trust the space made sacred by our intention. Now take three deep breaths. Inhale and exhale. As you exhale, take the thought, "I release all fear of this inner journey." Repeat this thought on the next two exhalations. Breathe in... breathe out. "I release all fear of this inner journey." And so, the journey begins.

I'd like you to visualize a long path that stretches before you. It may be a place known to you or it may be a new terrain. It may pass through a dark wood or across high mountains. At some point, you see before you an ancient iron gate. The gate is locked and vines cover it. You reach deep into your pocket and find a key. The key is large and rather heavy. Place the key into the lock, turning it in a complete circle so that the gate swings open. Now take another deep breath releasing any residue of fear, and walk through the open gate.

You find yourself now in a garden. It might be an English garden or perhaps a Japanese Zen garden with stone lanterns and tranquil pools of water with white lotus and gentle koi fish. Or any garden of your choice. See it. The flowers are in bloom. The smells intoxicate, causing you to smile. Just ahead is a house, which you recognize as the house of your dreams. You know this house for it is your very Self. Take a moment and visualize your house.

The door is locked but you hold in your hand the key. Visualize the key to your house and, taking a deep breath, open the door. Enter now and stand for a moment, taking in the profound feeling that you have come home. Then slowly yet with purpose, walk to your favorite room. Perhaps a paneled study lined with books of favorite authors. A fireplace glows providing warmth. Now walk to a large desk which overlooks the garden, and sit. After a moment, open the center drawer and take out paper and pen. See the pen that you will write with. Now look carefully at the virgin white page and honor it. But first, I'd like you to visualize your soul. It might be a bird or a butterfly or an animal, or a jewel or some other precious object. What would be a metaphor for your soul, your innermost being? See it. Experience it.

Now begin the dialogue. Visualize looking at your soul in whatever form it has chosen. Then ask it, soul, one single, simple question: "What do you want?"

This will not be the only or final answer for all time, simply the one soul gives you today, that is, now, this very moment.

For the next ten minutes — without undue thinking — open your eyes and begin the exercise, the Soul Dialogue. Simply write the question, "What do you want?" Then taking all the time you need, listen for soul's reply and write it down. Write it all down. There is no right answer. There is only your answer. Please begin now.

Listen. Make a way for yourself inside yourself.
Rumi

Jung and Individuation

During the First World War, Jung formed his principal psychological theories and archetypes, collective unconscious, and process of individuation. He transformed psychotherapy from a practice concerned primarily with treating the sick into a means for higher development of the personality. This approach would be called *analytical psychology*, a process of inner exploration that Jung would later call *individuation* — the goal being wholeness or realization of the Self.

After breaking from Sigmund Freud, Jung withdrew for a four-year retreat. During this time, he did little except to listen to his inner guide, which he named "Philemon." He drew pictures, paintings, and mandalas in what later became *The Red Book*. Jung wrote later in his autobiography, *Memories, Dreams, and Reflections*, that everything of value came from those four years of retreat, the foundation for all that was to come.

Jung did not care what others thought. He followed his inner guide and left a promising career with Freud to walk his own path. To the man who listens to his deepest Self, the world will surrender. And so it did.

Cultivating the Inner Voice

An important tool for staying in tune with your inner Self and in getting the most out of these exercises is to cultivate and deepen inner listening. Listening is more than simply recalling what you know. Over the years, though I have made my share of mistakes and wrong turns, I have learned to trust my inner voice — some may call it intuition. It is seldom wrong. All that is required is to be still and listen not to what the ego desires, but to the soul's calling. The voice, the signs, the turnings, the allies are always there — if we but listen. This voice may even save your life. Here is one example that happens to be a true story — my story.

I was twenty-something and living in New York City, earning my living then as an actress. An actress friend was visiting New York from Europe and invited me for tea at her hotel on Central Park South. When I walked into her room, my friend asked me to sit in a big chair by the window that overlooked Central Park. As soon as I sat there, I felt intensely uncomfortable, and could not explain why. A voice within told me quite distinctly to leave and to leave now as I was in danger. She began to serve tea, and after only ten minutes, I abruptly said, "I can't stay. I don't feel well." I hastily left and returned home. The minute I walked into my apartment, the phone rang. It was my friend, whose voice was trembling as she told me what had occurred soon after I left her.

"Do you remember that chair you were sitting on next to the window? Well, you'll never believe this, but a huge air conditioning unit on top of the building fell and crashed into that window and onto the chair where you were sitting! You might have been killed!"

Since that day, now decades ago, I have put full trust in that still, small voice within. It is far more valuable to me than my logical mind. Everyone has an intuitive capability if they take the time and intention to develop it. And it might even save your life!

EXERCISE

Think of a moment in your life when you listened to your intuitive or inner voice, and what happened because of it. Or recall a time when your intuitive voice was at odds with your logical mind. Which did you follow and what was the result? Write it down.

When you listen within, be prepared to make radical changes that family and friends may not always understand. Nonetheless, it is necessary to hold firm to what you know to be right for you.

EXERCISE

Remember a time you gave up something in order to follow your own inner voice. What was the result? Or a time when you didn't listen to your inner voice?

There are many ways to encourage your inner voice. One way is to be open to activities and collective events that encourage stillness and introspection — meditative retreats or workshops, for example, or silent group walks in nature, or Hatha yoga classes.

When you say yes to a night out, keep your radar alert that this is what will serve what is deepest in you. Discriminate. Say no to what doesn't serve. Here's one small example.

A friend of mine asked me to join him for a banquet that was dedicated to a good cause. I had also been told of another event that happened to be on the same evening. Some Bhutan Buddhist monks would be performing a healing ceremony. We would be asked to lie on the floor with closed eyes and listen to the healing chants. Part of me would have enjoyed going out with my friend on a dinner date at the banquet yet there was no contest. I had just returned from a week-long writers conference where I had taught two workshops and knew I needed the quiet, healing evening more.

EXERCISE

Think of a time you didn't listen to your inner voice and accepted to do something or go somewhere that was not the best thing for your deeper Self. Write about it and what was the result.

EXERCISE

Now remember a time you listened to your inner calling and said no to an invitation that did not feel right. Write about it and what was the result.

Once many years ago a relative chided me for going off to India for meditative retreats each year. She told me I was being selfish. I did not debate the accusation yet knew in my heart that it was not accurate. It was about values, priorities.

Her judgment made me consider though how my actions might seem to others — especially others who did not follow an inner call to wholeness. I came to understand how my years of seeking truth and acquiring various disciplines on the way to wholeness is the best work I could do — not only for my own journey but for others, as well. It made me a better friend and parent as well as a better teacher. To serve ego may well be a selfish act. To serve the Self, never.

> *It is returning, at last it is coming home to me — my own self and those parts of it that have long been abroad and scattered among all things and accidents.*
> Friedrich Nietzsche, *Thus Spoke Zarathustra*

Listen within, discriminate, and choosing will become easier. It is important to make sure we are living our lives and not experiencing our lives living us. We've all heard the saying, "Are you a human doing or a human being?" Naturally, we are both, but balance is essential. Sometimes another saying may help guide the way:

> *When in doubt, don't just do something.*
> *Sit.*

Chapter Five

Focused Journaling: A Powerful and Transformational Mirror

———

How do I know about the world?
By what is within me.
Lao Tzu

Every day the world is changed by ordinary people. A black woman refuses to sit at the back of a bus in Alabama. A young Chinese student stands stolidly in front of a tank in Tiananmen Square. In the distant Himalayas in India, there are meditating yogis who never leave their caves, yet some say that these wise ones are helping to keep the world in balance. Never underestimate the value of ordinary human beings, for they are the ones who change our world.

For all we know, it may do the world a greater service simply to discover who we are, one individual at a time. Courage is needed to face who we are, and to become aware of the repercussions of our existence on ourselves, our loved ones, and the world we inhabit. Accepting our own individual shadow or dark side and integrating it on the way to wholeness may well be the most important job as a human being.

Focused journaling is one tool to do just this. Ordinary journaling or automatic writing is writing whatever pops into your head, while focused journaling is directing a laser beam onto your psyche. To think of it in another way, it is looking directly at your Self and mirroring what you think and feel about how you view the world, specific subjects, events, and people.

As man evolved, the unknown was stripped of its mystery and the known replaced the unknown through the power of language. From awareness followed expressions of that awareness: the healing power of words. Creative expression can fill this long-neglected hole thereby returning us to who we truly are. To think of it another way, focused journaling is a creative inner dialogue with one's Self.

Creativity as Therapy

Creativity is not for the privileged few, but rather is a choice that anyone can make. It is a way of perceiving. These new exercises will tap the creative juices necessary to express yourself in any of the existing forms of art, and make you feel more alive than ever before. And, feeling alive is much more than mere survival.

> *Creativity is bringing forth something that the world has never seen before... creativity is the model for the original life.*
> Joseph Campbell

Joseph Campbell once remarked that unless a mythology is able to give its adherents a direct experience of the mystery of existence... mythology is not performing its most essential function. What outmoded myth are you living today?

Reading and healing have an age-old association. In ancient Egypt, libraries were known as *psyches iatreion*, "sanatoriums of the soul." During the Renaissance, the poetry of the Psalms was thought to banish vexations of the soul. Now, science has discovered what readers and writers have long known: words can help us heal and revitalize our bodies as well as our minds. And as a result, *bibliotherapy* — reading specific texts in response to particular situations or conditions — is becoming more and more popular among psychologists, physicians, and teachers. There is also a new field in psychology called *narrative psychology*, which looks at how human beings deal with experience by constructing stories and listening to the stories of others. What we think or read influences us because thought is powerful — both positively and negatively. What food are you putting inside your mind? To think creatively or outside the box activates a part of the brain that might otherwise lie dormant. In such ways, we can self-heal from within.

> *It's not what you look at that matters.*
> *It's what you see.*
> Henry David Thoreau

It is only by honoring your own point of view or perspective that you can express or share anything of lasting value. Some of us may have been discouraged from being subjective in school or even at home. Perhaps it is time to honor that inner voice. We have a duty to our deeper Self to be true to who and what we are. How to find your voice? By being still, turning within, and listening to that deeper Self.

Often the hardest part of focused journaling is simply sitting down. Be honest. Be bold. Know your Self. Honor your uniqueness yet understand that each individual is unique in different ways. Begin a journey of exploration by looking back at your own life.

To know what you want, you must first know who you are. By knowing yourself, you can better understand the world — as well as others. People change largely because they want different things at different times and ages. Desire forms what we are, and not only motivates what we do, but also what we don't do.

> *You are what your deepest desire is,*
> *As you desire, so is your intention.*
> *As your intention, so is your will.*
> *As is your will, so is your deed.*
> *As is your deed, so is your destiny.*
>
> The Upanishads

EXERCISE

Take a moment now. Close your eyes then breathe deeply. When you answer the following questions, don't think too long. Just go with what arises in the moment. Write the questions down then your responses by listening within.

Write responses to the following:

At age 12, I wanted to be a _____ because

_____.

At age 21, I wanted to be a _____ because

_____.

At age 31, I wanted to be a _____ because

_____.

At age 41, I wanted to be a _____ because

_____.

Today I choose to be a _____ because

_____.

Notice how what you thought to be true has changed over the years.

EXERCISE

- For this exercise, look at your responses to the exercise you just completed and focus on what about you has remained the same. Write a few lines about what within you has remained a constant.

- Now imagine a metaphor for that unchanging part of you. A bird? Plant? Tree? Animal? A family heirloom?

- Write about whatever associations arise.

EXERCISE

An individual is defined by what he desires and how he goes about obtaining that desire. Take three pages and put a name of a person you know on top of each page. First try to visualize each one, what he looks like, the expression in his eyes. Write in the first person from this friend or relative's point of view. Walk in his shoes. If you don't know the specifics, simply imagine them.

Part 1: In the first person, as if you are this person, write what you desire, then what you did to achieve that desire, as well as the price paid for following your dream or desire.

Part 2: Now go back and read what you have written. Try to suspend judgment. Simply listen to this person's story and see from his perspective. What do you *feel* as you do this? What comes up?

Part 3: Now jot down your own response to what this person says. Again, write in the first person, as if you are talking directly to this person.

Values as a Guiding Force

I write in order to discover myself.
Maya Angelou

While desire is a motivating drive in our lives, what we value serves as a guiding force. Take sufficient time to ponder the next questions.

EXERCISE

- What do you most respect in others?

- What makes you angry?

- What are you most curious about?

- What do you know to be true?

- If you could do anything in the world, what would you do first?

Transforming Negative to Positive

During the Middle Ages, scientists and philosophers studied alchemy. They reasoned that if they could discover a way to turn base metal into gold then they might discover the secret of life and the universe. One form of alchemy is discovering how to shift perspective and turn a negative situation into a positive one.

EXERCISE

For the following topics, the challenge is to transpose a negative situation or feeling into a positive one. Even if the situation and effect on you was not positive, try to discover something that made you grow in a certain way. If nothing in you responds to a topic, simply move on to the next. Don't feel you must do them all today. Take your time, contemplate then write down each response, allowing it to be as long as it needs to be.

• Something you gave to someone that was not appreciated.

• Being sick in bed.

• Where you would fly today if you could.

• What you strongly believe in.

• What you are no longer sure of.

• The moment you knew something had ended.

- What you wish you could still do.

- Something you treasure more than anything.

- Memories of eating chocolate or something else you love to eat.

- Feeling homesick.

- Feeling homesick for somewhere you have never been.

- An ideal day experienced.

- An ideal day imagined.

- What do you identify with in order to be who you are? Your job? Another person? A place? A role you play regularly?

- A selfish fear.

- An old dream.

- A marriage proposal.

- Making the bed.

- Scolding a child or being scolded when a child.

It is easier to forget in the rush of life that what we think or feel or visualize is the first important step toward actualization. So it matters tremendously what we hold in our minds. This reminds me of the Sage telling his disciple to meditate so many hours daily, only to be sure not to think of monkeys. Later, of course, the poor acolyte confessed that all he could think of was monkeys! So try not to create monkeys in your life. Allow sufficient time to be still and sink within to a deeper plateau. Sacred music can help or you may prefer silence.

This process of listening to the unconscious is greatly aided by recording your dreams, which often serve as a guide.

The Power of Dreams

I see visions which I could not see with my ordinary eye.
Maxine Hong Kingston, *Woman Warrior*

Like creativity, dreams arise from the unconscious. We have to create an empty space in our conscious minds for the unconscious to emerge with its varied gifts. All too often, conditioning prods one to rush in with interpretative meaning, learned meanings, which may serve only to flatten the true value of what arises naturally from within. Mental understanding won't necessarily change us. To be transformed requires something more than rational thinking. The conditioned way of mental knowing often strengthens the ego at the expense of soul. In fact, mere mental understanding may be overrated today. Marc Chagall said of his paintings that he didn't understand them at all. "They are only pictorial arrangements of images that obsess me." Thinking — though a valuable tool — is only handmaiden to a deeper process. As American novelist Willa Cather once remarked, "It is the inexplicable presence of the thing not named... "

The unconscious is an ally — if we listen. "The dream," said Jung, "is a little hidden door in the innermost and most secret recesses of the soul." Sigmund Freud called dreams "the royal road to the unconscious." Our dreams are written in the symbolic language of the unconscious.

Sometimes you wake up from a dream and the emotions are vivid and clear. Other times the feelings come in images like paintings, where you have to put yourself in that world and intuit their meaning before you uncover the feelings. Images can be more powerful than mere words. They speak in metaphor. And metaphor is the language of the soul. Well-chosen images can help us integrate mind and feeling, which in today's culture have been split asunder. Metaphor or symbolic image is a shortcut to revealing what you are trying to express or need to hear. It is through metaphor that the process of life and art can be seen as in a mirror. Look for metaphors in both waking and dream states. Awaken that part of the mind that generates images. Let each image invade you, feel it, note whatever associations arise, then write with your senses, feelings, and invisible wonderings. Let intuition guide. Write what will nourish the soul.

The visionary is the only true realist.
Federico Fellini

Even when the details of a dream elude you, often a definite mood lingers. If nothing else, record the feeling or mood you are left with upon awakening. It is a good idea to keep a journal or notebook handy next to your bed in order to record what comes through.

EXERCISE

Create the habit of asking for guidance from "dream knowing." Before sleep, ask the guides what you wish to know. Perhaps you are in a life transition and unsure of the next turning in your journey. Ask. If no answer arises the next morning, ask again and yet again. Be open to what comes and what symbols appear. Write down whatever comes. Do the same in your daily meditation. Be on the lookout for what appears in your mail, a phone call from an old friend, or a stranger you happen to meet. The Divine works in many ways.

Remember this joke? A man believes in God. A flood arises and he is drowning yet not worried, knowing that God will save him. A young man in a rowboat comes and says to him, "Swim over here." The man shakes his head, saying, "No, I don't need you. God will save me." Then a helicopter hovers overhead and yells at him to take the ladder. The man shakes his head again, saying, "No need, God will save me." Well, you probably have already guessed what happens next. The man drowns. When he gets to heaven, he confronts God, saying, "I believed in you all my life. I believed that you would save me from drowning and yet you did not." God replies, "I did try to save you twice. I sent a young man in a rowboat and later I sent a helicopter, but you said no." Similarly, your answer may not come in the way you expect, but it will come in its own language and in its own time — not yours or mine.

EXERCISE

Once you have recorded a dream, set aside some time in order to work it. First be still and meditate on the meaning of the dream and any associations, and then listen to whatever arises. Listen without interpretation. If you don't see anything clearly, invite the unconscious to tell you more about this particular dream before going to sleep.

EXERCISE

Using the dream from the preceding exercise, write a monologue or dialogue from each dream character's point of view, whether that character is an animal or a person. Probe what the characters feel as well as what they are trying to say. As Jung reminds, don't forget that all the characters in your dream symbolize some aspect of yourself.

Lessons from the Past

From time to time, it is helpful to remember what the past has taught us. However, as memory is subjective, it is rarely an accurate account of what has actually transpired. It is selective. Memory is, more than anything, about perspective — not facts.

EXERCISE

• Think back to a time you experienced as a turning point in your life. Be specific. What would be a metaphor for this period of your life? Perhaps an animal, a natural disaster, or some other collective event, or some physical object may come to mind. Visualize the metaphor. Write it down then write whatever associations arise. Trust the process. It is not necessary to know where it is taking you.

• Now choose one simple, specific memory that reminds you — even now — of that time. It might be a certain food or glass of wine, a storm, a song, a gift, a tree, etc. Stick to this small detail and allow it to lead you on. Know that it is not necessary to know where it is taking you. Just follow your vision of what happened, any and all associations, and how you felt about it at the time. Keep writing. Be ruthlessly honest.

• Now compare this with how you look upon it all now. What did you learn? Did this period in your life change you in some fundamental way — for better or worse?

The Inevitable Impulse to Self-Express

On Sunday, December 18, 1994, Jean-Marie Chauvet led his two friends, Éliette Brunel and Christian Hillaire, on the Cirque d'Estre toward the cliffs in southern France. A faint air current emanating from a small opening at the end of a small cave had attracted his attention and he now wanted to satisfy his curiosity once and for all. All three had a passion for speleology and had long stopped counting their discoveries. It was late in the afternoon and the small cavity into which they penetrated was already known since it was situated very close to a popular hiking trail. But there, behind the fallen rocks, they were sure there was something more. They dug a passage, crawled through it, and soon found themselves at the edge of an obscure shaft. They did not have the equipment necessary to continue. By the time they got back to their cars, night had already fallen. They gathered up the essential tools, hesitated for a moment, and then returned to their discovery. They descended with their speleological ladder and discovered a vast chamber with a very high ceiling. They progressed in a single-file line toward another chamber as big as the first one, and there admired the unexpected geological wonders that surrounded them. They also saw animal bones scattered on the floor. They explored almost the entire network of chambers and galleries, and on the way back out, Éliette saw an amazing sight in the beam of her lamp: a small mammoth drawn with red ochre on a rocky spur hanging from the ceiling. "They were here!" she cried out, and from that instant they began searching all of the walls with great attention. They discovered hundreds of paintings and engravings. Perhaps they were more fluent in the language of the unconscious than we are today.

The Chauvet Caves in southern France were discovered in 1994. German filmmaker Werner Herzog did a fine documentary film, *Cave of Forgotten Dreams* (2010), about these caves and their paintings, which date as far back as 35,000 years. Even then, the Neanderthal cave painters were inspired to leave something of themselves behind them, something for future men to see.

Apart from the impressive animal cave paintings, I was especially struck by the imprints of the artist's hands, palm down, that were painted on the cave walls. Hand stencils were created by blowing red pigments onto a hand placed against the wall as if the Neanderthal artist were signing his or her name. What is this impulse to self-express, to create, to leave one's mark upon the future? Whatever it was 35,000 years ago, it is still here with us today. It lies within each of us.

What would you choose to leave behind?

EXERCISE

If you could leave anything behind as a kind of legacy to your life on earth, what would it be? Remember the imagination is without limits. Write about what your legacy would be.

*This, then, is the power of myth: to
awaken the psyche to wonder at the
universe and to the creative life.*
  Joseph Campbell

The individual has an experience of his own in which he
seeks to communicate through signs; and if his realization
has been of a certain depth and import, his communication
will have the value and force of living myth.

The Power of Choice

Remember that there is always choice. For this next
focused journaling exercise, throw the windows of your
mind wide open, allowing yourself complete freedom as
you imagine the answers to the following:

EXERCISE

If I could live anywhere in the world, I would
live _____ because _____.

If I could do anything I wanted to, I would
_____ because _____.

If I could be with anyone I choose, I would live
with _____ because _____.

EXERCISE

Repeat the same exercise. Remember that before action are thought and vision. Hold the dream in your mind and in your heart. It might just surprise you what can happen!

If I could live anywhere in the world, I would live _____ because _____.

If I could do anything I wanted to, I would _____ because _____.

If I could be with anyone I choose, I would live with _____ because _____.

EXERCISE

Now note what came up differently and write about why you think your answers shifted.

Never forget that the power of choice is ever there. Even if we cannot always control outer events in our lives, the one choice that remains is to choose our perspective.

The late psychiatrist Viktor Frankl, in *Man's Search for Meaning*, shares his story of being a Holocaust survivor during World War II. After witnessing his entire family killed in a concentration camp, Frankl had an epiphany that not only changed his life but became the foundation of his important work later in New York. He was stripped of everything and everyone who held meaning for him. Then he was stripped of any power to change the horror around him. Then Frankl realized that though he had no power over outer events, he did have power over how he perceived what was happening. Frankl later wrote, "When we are no longer able to change a situation, we are challenged to change ourselves." This shift in perspective determined his life from then on and helped hundreds of his patients.

In other words, we can choose how we view what is happening to us. Remember that before action, comes thought and vision. Hold the vision in your mind and in your heart, and it might surprise you what happens!

> *Whatever you can do, or dream you can, begin it.*
> *Boldness has genius, power and magic in it.*
> *Begin it now.*
>   Johann Wolfgang von Goethe

Chapter Six

Integrating the Opposites: Standing in the Light, Facing the Dark

Where the light is brightest, the shadows are deepest.

Johann Wolfgang von Goethe

Exploring and integrating the polarities that live within can release creative and healing energies. Jung wrote extensively of the "tension of opposites." Each person is a synthesis of contradictory attitudes and possesses opposing traits. Jung describes how this inner tension creates movement in our lives. According to Jung, an archetype or mythic prototype remains dormant until its opposite is aroused. Then it is activated and the energy generated between them creates a *third*, i.e., *tertium quid*. That is, something new is born from that tension. This third is the life or story produced from a dance of the opposites. Without this tension of opposites or pull, there would be no creativity, no life, and certainly no potential of transformation.

*Taking it in its deepest sense, the shadow is
the invisible saurian tail that man still drags
behind him. Carefully amputated, it becomes
the healing serpent of the mysteries.*
C. G. Jung

Both healing and growth come through working and integrating the shadow side within all of us. No one is purely good or bad. The fact is our opposing selves are like the two wolves fighting in our hearts. Yes, it depends on which one you feed yet you cannot simply ignore the darker voice within. The shadow side must be heard and acknowledged for you to learn, integrate, and move on. By going through and beyond your own story, you will connect to the great universal story of us all, for in the specific lies the universal. What in your history, both positive and negative, made you who you are today?

*There are some things you learn best in calm,
and some in storm.*
Willa Cather

EXERCISE

Describe two turning points in your life: one which arose from a positive event, another from a negative event. Add what lesson was learned from both.

While each of us has a positive inner voice that calls us toward the light, we usually have a negative inner voice as well. It pays to listen to both. This negative inner voice is most often an internalized critical parent. We cannot just pretend that this darker voice is not sounding any more than we can disavow what family we were born into. We can only work with what we have and become the very best of who we are meant to be. This is growth — not simplistic pretending to be someone or something else.

For instance, in my own life, I rebelled against a conservative Texas family and chose early on to live thousands of miles away from where I grew up. Creatively, politically, and spiritually, I felt there was little in common with where I came from. However, looking back now, I am grateful. The conservative, prudent genes in me have helped me to survive a freelance career in the arts. Also I was bred on solid values and the importance of responsibility, hard work, and compassion for others less fortunate. I recognize now that soul knew exactly what it was doing to place me in Texas, after all. Even the rebellious spirit that arose in that environment strengthened me for the battles yet to come, living and working in New York and Hollywood. Soul can be trusted. It knows its job.

Seizing my life in your hands, you thrashed it clean
On the savage rocks of Eternal Mind.
How its colors bled, until they grew white!
You smile and sit back; I dry in your sun.
Rumi (translated by Andrew Harvey)

It is important to accept those parts of us that are like our parents — especially those traits that we may not like. In Jung's autobiography, *Memories, Dreams, and Reflections*, Jung admits to his worst trait of being obstinate. Yet, he also says, that without this trait, he would not have achieved what he achieved in his life.

Sometimes negative traits can have positive outcomes. Anger, for example, can help you to get in touch with feelings, overcome repression, and even change the world for the better.

> *Under heaven all can see beauty as beauty*
> *only because there is ugliness. All can know*
> *good as good only because there is evil.*
> *Therefore having and not having arise together.*
> Lao Tse, *Tao Te Ching*

For instance, on one side, I have a strong tendency to withdraw from the world and contemplate spiritual truths. On the opposite side, I have an equally strong desire to self-express through acting and writing plays, movies, and books, as well as teaching. One side surrenders the world and the other lives in the world of creative expression. For years, my life would be like a pendulum swinging back and forth following these two opposite selves, creating a continous inner tension. I would act or have a play produced in the theatre in New York. When success and money came, I would fly to India and retreat for months. Eventually, I would return and pick up my career again. However, I began to notice that I felt most deeply myself when I was allowing self-expression and that this, at least for me, was a true *sadhana* or spiritual practice.

Perhaps we serve soul most by being deeply who we are and doing what we are meant to do. In an earlier chapter, I spoke of dharma and how it is better to be a good servant than a bad king. This means to delve within and honestly discover what it is you are meant to do in this life. This perspective gives more weight than simply choosing a career. Indeed, one's dharma may be being a wife or mother as well as any other vocation. One is not superior to another as long as it is true to who you are.

At some point, it became clear to me that spiritual life was not either/or but both/and. So it was not a case of living in the world or withdrawing from it at all. The challenge then was to integrate the two parts of myself. Later as a playwright and screenwriter — as well as university professor — I committed to writing only consciousness-raising stories and to inspire others to explore what stories lay deep within them. Somehow a spiritual thread ran through whatever I wrote. It was clearly shown to me that the whole of life is meditation — even writing. So the challenge was not in choosing which side to follow, but rather integrating both tendencies in a singular journey toward wholeness. The opposing pull between these two sides became the movement to manifest thus integrating both life and purpose. Creating was my way of being in the world — if not of it.

EXERCISE

Often the opposites within seem to be at war. Write down traits seen as negative that prevent you from creating the space to tap your creative potential or walk your path. Then, go down the list and see which items are rational-based, which are fear-based, and, perhaps, which are a bit of each.

Dare to change. All true things must change, and only that which changes remains true.
Friedrich Nietzsche

There is another factor at play today. We live long. Did you know that during the Middle Ages, the standard life span was only thirty-six years? We live so long that today many lives are lived in this one life. It thereby becomes important to be open to change. This may mean more than one marriage, more than one residence, and often more than one career. Change is life and growth. Forms are made to dissolve. There are always new parts of our selves that wait to be discovered. However, when it is time for a shift, sometimes we may not heed the subtle message for change. This will often manifest as someone or something giving us a jolt to wake us up to the needed change.

For instance, I had felt for three years that my New York life had ended. Yet I stayed on. I was returning from a Fulbright year in India when a former student, to whom I had entrusted my apartment, had locked me out with the aim of taking over the apartment for herself. Of course, I was shocked by the betrayal and to what lengths another may go in order to find a great apartment in the city — and yes, it was a great apartment! Later, I remembered Jung had said that if you don't listen to the needs of the unconscious, a situation will rise up and bump you. This was such a situation. I gave up the apartment (though I made sure the treacherous student did not get it) and moved to Hollywood, something I had considered doing for three years. So this wayward student became the vehicle I needed to take the next step of my journey. The move launched a new career and a happier life. Often a seeming calamity is an angel in disguise.

> *My barn having burned down,*
> *I can now see the moon.*
> Zen saying

It helps to be alert when one life is ending so that we may embrace the next. Daily meditation can help us lead a more centered, more aware life.

EXERCISE

Take ten minutes each morning and sit in the same place daily. It might begin by taking deep breaths or simply sitting with closed eyes and visualizing something peaceful or something loved. After a while, this will become habit and a necessary way to begin your day.

Once my twelve-year-old son was late for school and ran out of our thirty-seventh-floor apartment (yes, the one we later lost in New York before moving to California). Two minutes later, he was back, saying, "I forgot to do my meditation." I smiled as this was said in the same manner as "I forgot to brush my teeth." Meditation was a daily habit in our home, considered as important — if not more important — as brushing teeth.

Embracing change is often frightening and yet without change, we do not grow. What small voices or hints do you hear or feel from your unconscious? Something within will usually provide a clue if we are listening. If we are not listening, then usually we may expect to be shaken when still living a part of our life that has completed soul's purpose.

EXERCISE

- What voices in the past did you not listen to until something rose up and gave you a bump? Write down your response now.

- What about now? Is soul giving you clues as to some change that is needed in your life? Take a moment now and write them down.

- Ask yourself if you are living the life that is right for you at this time. Or are you living the life someone else wishes you to live that may not be in sync with your soul's purpose? Write it. Write it all down.

The Blame Game

That which is to give Light must endure burning.
Viktor Frankl, *Man's Search for Meaning*

Whose fault is it if we are not living a true life? One woman may say, "I wish I could be free, but I must take care of my aging parent." Another husband or wife may say, "I want my husband or wife to be happy so I'm doing this job even though I hate it." "My father always wanted me to be a doctor like he was." "It would kill my parents if I followed my bliss." There are so many voices that can keep one from not following his or her dream. Sometimes of course there are legitimate reasons why walking our path may be delayed. Delay need not mean abandoning our dreams though. Often we may imagine voices of those around us in order to serve our own fear of change or risk, and of following a new path.

EXERCISE

At the top of a page, make two headings for two separate columns: "Legitimate Reason" and "Fear Speaking." Now list something you have desired or dreamed of doing for some while yet hesitated. There may be legitimate reasons not to do something as well as blockages caused by fear. Discern which heading applies.

It is sometimes true that when following our inner voice, others close to us may be hurt, temporarily. Yet I have found that if we are true to ourselves and walk our walk, the universe supports us and even those around us in the end. Families tend to forgive happy, fulfilled human beings and like being around them, too! What may seem like selfishness is booty for all in the end. The inner guide is a deeper voice and not selfish as some think, but one which, in time, serves the whole. Granted, it is an act of faith to listen within then to act on that inner guidance. By this, I don't simply mean the ego desire of the moment. The truth is, with rare exceptions, there is usually only one person to blame for not living our dream or following the inner voice.

Often those parts of us that are repressed or hidden from our consciousness may be projected onto another or onto a group of people. A friend of mine is forever disparaging the rich without taking into account that they, too, are each individuals. The shadow of our times is an increasing emphasis on the collective, overlooking the individual.

The same principle holds true on the personal level as well. Virtually every projection forms a relationship within our psyche. It is this relationship — both positive and negative — that will reveal something meaningful to you if you are aware. Cultivate the habit of noticing when you project some judgment upon another and investigate if this in any way relates to something you may have repressed in yourself.

Keeping a journal and recording projections as they arise can hasten the inner work of integration. In writing down experiences, try to capture your thoughts, feelings, and actions in as much immediate detail as possible. Projections often resist coming to the surface of conscious awareness. They are best teased out by attending to details.

EXERCISE

Remember a time when an incident or person may have pushed a button creating a strong reaction within.

- Exactly what did the other person say that triggered you?
- What part of it had the most impact upon you?
- What feelings arose? Bodily sensations?
- Fantasies of what you would like to do or say to that person?
- Think about the aspect of "you" that was so affected. This part of the Self will gradually reveal its own nature and desires more clearly.

The more each individual can own his or her shadow or repressed parts, the more it is possible to attract more positive energies into your life.

EXERCISE

Feed or visualize positive thoughts as the fuel that powers your goals. Make a list of two columns with two headings: "Negative" and "Positive." Under Negative, list any negative thoughts or feelings you have lived with and are now willing to release. Under Positive, list a new version transposed from the Negative version. After completing the list of both, read them and decide which ones you will choose to adopt.

> *Wherever you go, there you are.*
> Zen saying

If we're honest, the main problem in life is simply ourselves. I have a friend who has spent years travelling the globe in order to find the perfect place to live. He flies to Bali then New Zealand then Ecuador and on and on, always returning, never having found the perfect spot. I finally told my friend, "You know the truth is there is no perfect place for the simple reason that wherever we go, we take ourselves with us. And as we are not perfect, the 'where' will not be either."

Your real Self has no hiding place no matter where you go. Live in Self and the place will find you. Live in Self and wherever you are will be home. This applies as well to finding the perfect mate.

Dare to be Vulnerable

Dare to let go of control and open to your own vulnerability. Often when we're hurt, we no longer trust vulnerability and we create the habit of numbing ourselves as a way of self-protection. The thing is though, when you numb yourself or build a wall of defense, nothing gets through. It shuts you down and love, joy, a sense of adventure, etc., are also blocked. Love makes us vulnerable as it must do.

Novelist William Styron underwent a severe depression, and wrote a courageous book about his struggles, *Darkness Visible: A Memoir of Madness*. He exorcised his dark demon. I last saw William Styron at a chamber music concert in New York, and a gentler and more kindly man I have never met. Kind men may sometimes harbor the darkest of demons. Anyone on a committed inner path must at some time, in some way, face the demon or shadow within. Be clear that the shadow's home is within, not without. Face your shadow and do the necessary inner work and Light will find you. Even breakdowns can be opportunities for a spiritual breakthrough.

> *The best way out is always through.*
> Robert Frost

EXERCISE

* Visualize a metaphor (animal, bird, archetype, or object) that represents your dark side. Face your shadow in whatever form arises then ask the question, "What is the dark shadow side of my soul?" Write this question at the top of the page then listen to its response. Write down whatever comes — without judgment.

* After you have finished transcribing this message from the dark side, repeat this sentence as though it is a mantra: "I accept this part of myself without judgment. Though I choose to stand in the light, I will listen to the voice of my shadow and learn."

* Finally write down what you feel you have learned in life by embracing your own dark side.

> *I am, you anxious one.*
> *Don't you sense me, ready to break*
> *into being at your touch?*
> *My murmurings surround you like shadowy wings.*
> *I am the dream you are dreaming.*
> *When you want to awaken, I am waiting.*
>   Rainer Maria Rilke

The Perils of Idealism

Another aspect that arises on the journey is reality versus illusion. Discrimination is needed in order not to impose or project perfection on another or even on ourselves.

Idealism is something I have always been prey to, as far back as I can remember. To have ideals may aid us in setting high goals for life and work. This is good. And yet to live with too much idealism may sometimes invite disillusionment in its wake. To expect life or work or a life partner to be ideal makes it difficult to accept or appreciate what is.

Amor Fati (Love What Is)

Loving and accepting what is can be the ticket to moving more smoothly through life and love. Though ideals may have their place in honoring our goals and challenges, if they overtake what realistically can be, they sometimes may fail us in the end.

Of course, the buck stops here. First, we idealize who we think we should be — and sometimes this creates unnecessary obstacles. Perhaps you may have seen a quote on a card that reads, "Super Woman (I have no choice)." This is a humorous comment on an ideal birthed by the feminist movement in America in the seventies and eighties. Thousands of women bought this and the myth of super woman continues to this day. The idea is that a single woman can and should do it all: marriage, children, and profession. Of course, it is right that women finally have the opportunities to marry, mother, and have careers. It is prudent, however, to be kind to ourselves and ask for help when needed, and not identify too keenly with being perfect.

Often my habit is to push myself even now as I did in my twenties. Though my mind thinks I'm still twenty-eight, my body — now decades older — does not necessarily follow. Hence, I push until struck down with a mighty flu, which entitles me to complete rest — without self-judgment. Balance needs to be observed — even practiced. And for a good life, there must be a balance of work and rest. (I'm not only talking to you here. I'm talking to myself!)

It is important to remember that the aim is growth of the soul toward wholeness — not perfection. All too often one is taken for the other. There is no absolute perfection on the phenomenal level, and to think otherwise is to follow an illusive ideal. By integrating the light and dark aspects of ourselves through nonjudgmental awareness, we are on the way to wholeness.

> *The outer event becomes metaphor to the inner world of the psyche.*
> Alice O. Howell, *Jungian Synchronicity in Astrological Signs and Ages*

While the so-called New Agers have contributed some worthy aspects in the last few decades, they have, in my opinion, also created new problems, most prominently that of over-simplistic thinking. For instance, many advocate that if you only think positive thoughts then all will go well in your life, all the time. No illness, no accidents, no breakups or breakdowns, and so on. I feel something very close to anger when I meet someone suffering with cancer who is not only dealing with the disease but with the acquired mindset that she has caused the illness by not thinking positively enough! A bumper sticker I once saw proclaimed, "Shit Happens" and so it does. Life is a package deal, which means a bit of both darkness and light.

It is not what happens to us that is important, but what we make of it. While we cannot always control outer events, we can opt how to *perceive* what is happening to us. And this shift in perspective can make things better. If we focus on the Light, then the effect of whatever happens eventually contributes to our common good.

It takes a certain degree of courage to see ourselves as we are and not through a rose-colored lens. Courage is needed to see ourselves as we are at each step of the journey. Negative traits are there to spur growth, and deserve our attention. They move us toward transformative discovery.

Jung once remarked, "Thank God for our neuroses!" By this, he meant that this is how we learn and are forced to grow.

*The moment you accept that this is the way it is,
the transformation has begun.*
   John O'Donohue

Chapter Seven

A Shamanic Journey: Communicating with Spirit and Ancestral Guides

---

*Life began for me when I ceased to admire
and began to remember.*
Willa Cather

Once in East Africa, Bill Moyers sat alone on the shores of an ancient lake, and it suddenly struck him what community is. It is gathering around a fire and listening to another share his story. Imagine as you experience this chapter, that you are sitting around an ancient fire and sharing your story.

A Nod to the Ancestors

I had just returned from teaching *The Way of Story* workshop at Far Horizons, located in the Sequoia National Park in California. At an altitude of over seven thousand feet, a group of women met for five days in a rustic setting amidst the towering sequoia trees. No electricity, no cell phones, no email. It was a perfect setting to turn inward and share our stories creating a community. On the last evening, I arranged for a ritual fire to be built and asked the workshop participants to prepare an offering for the fire. They collected pinecones, branches, leaves, and worked with paints, paper, cloth, and glue to create a work of art worthy of a ritual fire sacrifice. I reminded them that it is the intention behind the ritual that gives it the power. Just before dark, I led them in a visualization and Soul Dialogue so that whatever arose within could be spoken to the fire at the time of their offerings.

While we stood in a circle around the great fire, I asked them to close their eyes then simply call out the country or countries their ancestors came from. Then I asked the ancestor spirits to encircle us as we continued the fire ritual. It was a powerful reminder that we are not alone.

It is necessary not to forget that we come from a long line of ancestors, and to offer them our thanks. Let us begin this chapter by offering a ritual to our ancestors.

EXERCISE

- List those ancestors you know or simply name the countries or cultural tribes that are your forebears.

- With pen and ink or pastels, draw symbols of your cultural background. For instance, I might draw a Celtic labyrinth or spiral with certain words in that language.

- You might wish to make something from sticks and leaves or seaweed. A full moon would be a good time or whenever it feels right.

- Use a fire pit or fireplace and meditate first expressing your gratitude for the long line of ancestors who brought you to now. Ask them for guidance. Then bow and offer your token as a sacrifice to the fire.

- If a dream comes later this night, record it, and work the dream, thus integrating your ancestral line to live on in you as spirit guides.

Sometimes the spirit of an ancestor you never knew may be an influence in your own life whether you are aware of this or not. You carry their genes as well.

EXERCISE

- Hold a photo or painting of an ancestor you've never met.

- What speaks to you about this photo or painting?

- Imagine what he or she was like, his or her story.

- Where did your ancestor live? Perhaps go to Google Earth to help you imagine what it was like there.

- Print out pictures of where your ancestor came from along with photographs of family members no longer living and make a collage.

- Ask for your ancestor's blessing.

Welcoming the Spirit Guides

There are more things in heaven and earth,
Horatio, than are dreamt of in your philosophy.
William Shakespeare, *Hamlet*

A few years ago, I was invited to a dinner by a trumpet player who was staying at the home of the director of Meditation Mount, a spiritual retreat in Ojai, California. My new Hungarian friend made dinner and we were joined by his friend, the director. I spoke of a fascinating book given to me the day before by an intuitive health practitioner who said, "I feel you are supposed to read this book." Later that night, mesmerized, I stayed up reading it to the end. The book was *Entering the Circle*, by Olga Kharitidi, M.D., a memoir relating her journey to Altai in Siberia and her unexpected encounter with a powerful shaman who changed her life. As we discussed earlier, shamans are those who bridge the real world and the invisible world, carrying messages to the collective from the other side. And the earliest shamans came from Siberia thousands of years ago.

Later when we finished dinner and were having tea, there was a knock on the door. The director answered and there on her doorstep stood an unusual looking man with a beard, and next to him, a young woman from Berkeley. Though unannounced, the unexpected strangers were invited in and the young woman translated from Russian what the unusual man began to tell us. "I come from Siberia and am travelling through North and South

America giving talks. I had not planned to come to this place but something drew me."

I spontaneously shared that the night before I had read an amazing book about an Altai shaman. The Siberian stranger looked at me with laughing eyes and said, "I am from that place." Here was a clear example of synchronicity. Synchronicity is a seemingly chance encounter or event that brings meaning, revealing an interconnection between the Self and the beyond.

Later that evening, he offered to perform a shamanic ritual. As we all sat in a circle, the mysterious shaman, wrapped in wolf skin, began to beat his drum. Then, possessed by his spirit guide, he began to sway to an ancient dance. Afterwards, still in trance, he came and stood before each of us and with piercing yet compassionate eyes, offered predictions about what would happen in our respective lives. Though he knew nothing of me beforehand, I was struck that he predicted I would a few years later write this book about healing and the effect it would one day have.

Synchronicities abound when one is on the inner path. I don't remember the Siberian shaman's name and probably will never see him again, yet some mysterious energy brought us all together that memorable evening. And the local health practitioner was a helper in the magic circle — even though she never met the shaman. Life is truly magical. In fact, more and more, I have come to view such occurrences as the norm.

The storyteller serves the story.
The fool serves the moment.
The shaman serves the tribe.
Tony Allen, Afro-beat drummer

Thank goodness for the Holy Fools, for in the moment is eternity!

Transmissions on the energetic level occur all the time, more so when we walk with open hearts and open minds. Once I was travelling with friends in Alaska, and I suddenly told my friend who was driving to stop the car. We were in the middle of nowhere in Wrangell-St. Elias National Park, the largest wilderness park in North America. He turned and looked at me questioningly, and I simply pointed outside the window to a large lynx with great eyes who was casually sitting by the road, watching us. For five minutes or so, we all sat in awe looking back at the wild lynx. I was struck that she showed no fear and remained seated while staring directly into my eyes. I felt something enter and knew that this transmission was a sacred, timeless moment to be honored — if not fully understood.

Creatives learn to value living in the unknown. Space is needed for magic to happen. Here is another example of synchronicity or meaningful coincidence where we may find ourselves experiencing reality on more than one plane.

A while back, I was having a series of shamanic dreams involving birds and animals. The owl dream, as

I refer to the most powerful dream, stayed with me for days and days as a kind of unseen presence. Though I cannot say what the full meaning of this particular dream was, I do know that it remains with me as a living presence or guide. (See Chapter 8 in my earlier book, *The Way of Story*, for a full account.) I dreamt of a large white owl three feet high, seven crows, and a white buffalo. The morning after this dream, it was reported in the news that a white buffalo — considered extremely rare and sacred to Native Americans — had been born in America.

However, the strongest presence in this dream, for me, was the three-foot-tall white owl standing to my right, offering a kind of energy transmission by gently staring at me. This owl became the focused dream image. Initially, I thought about all manner of owl associations, both personal and collective, and wrote these down, gathering knowledge of Minerva, the goddess of wisdom, and various Native American symbols. Then I took a quiet moment and simply sat with the image of the owl — without trying to analyze anything. From this arose a powerful *felt* sense of the owl. I sank deeper into myself, and felt the owl or owl-ness surround my entire body. I disappeared into the great owl yet retained my own form. Its spirit lay as a protective cover and poured into me. I became still, mind was no more, and the feeling of a mighty blessing overcame me. Energy as circles of light swirled in my heart chakra while a gentle tingling filled my whole body. Tears of gratitude and awe filled my eyes.

Jungian analyst and author James Hillman says, "To look at animals from an underworld perspective means to regard them as carriers of soul... there to help us see in the dark."

The morning after the owl dream, I hiked with a friend on Shelf Road overlooking the Ojai Valley in Southern California. Feeling someone or something looking at me, I stopped and turned around and there on a nearby branch in the middle of the day sat a small barn owl, staring directly at me. We stood staring for a while, then it flew off over my left shoulder as the dream owl had done the night before. Synchronicity. My friend said she had hiked on this road in town for twenty years and had never once seen an owl. After returning home from the hike, I wrote these words:

Silent wings, sharp beak,
Seer and hunter of the night.
Owl wisdom.

What was interesting to me was that I felt absolutely no need to understand the meaning of this experience. It was a gift to be received and honored. And this was more than enough.

Just when I'm in my corner writing all alone and feeling cut off from the outer world, something happens to remind me how interconnected we are — despite ourselves. Quite recently, I received a long, handwritten, and amazing letter from a Native American prisoner in Chaparral Prison in New Mexico, who had somehow found a copy of my book, *The Way of Story: The Craft & Soul of Writing.* Nathaniel is a descendent of Apache warriors, whose great-grandfather rode with Geronimo. Here are two small excerpts from his eleven-page letter:

"I was blessed to get hold of a copy of your most wonderful book, *The Way of Story.* I did the Soul Dialogue and this is what came. I want you to have it. Thank you once again. You are deserving of my deepest gratitude and praise."

Imprisoned for unintentionally killing his six-year-old daughter while driving while intoxicated, he writes of imagining he is an eagle soaring free: "I would love to just spread my wings on the highest branch overlooking the dark canyons and sense that there is nothing but a day of flight in store for me...."

Here is an example of using writing to tap into shamanic, healing spirits — in this case, the spirit of the eagle. In ways as these, ancient myths come alive and live through us today, guiding us, healing us. These stories are all examples of active allies: a Siberian shaman from Altai; a wild lynx in the Alaskan wilderness; a mighty owl in a dream; and Nathaniel's soaring eagle.

Community is formed through shared stories.
It's the history of our kindnesses
that alone makes this world tolerable.
   Robert Louis Stevenson

All four examples were unexpected, each a gift from the spirit realm. I have often noticed that the best moments of my life arise unasked for, and unexpected.

EXERCISE

- Think of an encounter you experienced in the waking state with a subtle guide in a seeming chance meeting with human or animal or bird. It should have a definite charge, quite different from other life encounters.

- Close your eyes and visualize it, remembering not only the details but the mood or feeling of it.

- Now write about it.

> *A single dream is more powerful than*
> *a thousand realities.*
> J. R. R. Tolkien, author of *Lord of the Rings*

EXERCISE

- Now think of a visitation you have experienced in a dream. Focus on a specific animal or figure in the dream and visualize not only the person, bird, or animal, but the feeling it evoked.

- Now begin to write. You might write it as a dialogue between the two of you. For instance, ask the figure what message it carries.

Let intuition guide. It quite often will be ever so much wiser than the logical left brain. Dare to open the portal and invite unknown allies.

> *Unless you accept inner adventure as a way of life, Discovery will not come to you.*
> Sri Nisargadatta Maharaj, *I Am That*

EXERCISE

- Stop reading and take a solitary walk, in some form of natural surroundings, if possible.

- Simply walk in search of a new metaphor for this time in your life. It might be a flower opening, a hummingbird searching for pollen, a cloud wandering aimlessly by, or a woodpecker industriously pecking away.

- When you return home, sit down, close your eyes, visualize and feel your chosen metaphor, then write about it, whatever associations arise, and what they mean to you today.

If you wish to change your life, change your metaphor. Metaphor is the language of the soul. Metaphor can be a symbolic image of what you and your life are about. It is through metaphor that the process of life and art can be seen as if in a mirror. Look for metaphors in both waking and dream states. Awaken that part of the mind that generates images. Well-chosen images can help us integrate thoughts and feelings, which in today's culture have been split asunder. Dare to explore the unknown regions of the psyche, for therein lies creative gold. And there, spirit allies dwell.

Unwanted Inner Voices

All too often whenever we sit quietly, negative voices sometimes arise in our mind — usually an inner parent or a more skeptical self. These are past conditionings or imprints we have carried for many years and which may continue unhealthy patterns in our daily life.

EXERCISE

* For now, simply listen to the negative voices in your mind. Identify them. Name them.

* Now begin a compassionate dialogue with them. Allow yourself to listen to what they have to say, then after thanking them for their contribution, gently tell them that you no longer need their input in your life.

* See them as uninvited guests in your home and now is the time for them to leave. Without anger or bitterness, bid them farewell. Know that if and when they revisit you, you will simply witness them as uninvited guests in your house.

* In my experience, the inner voices believe they are helping us or protecting us from disappointment

or some other negative outcome. They depart more easily if we acknowledge and thank them before letting them go.

Heavy Baggage

What is the heavy baggage you carry? It may be attachments or challenges of those we love. The responsibility of love can seem at times a heavy weight. It may be financial worries or difficulties in our work life.

If your heart was a suitcase, what color would it be? Would it be hard shell or soft? What would be inside the suitcase?

EXERCISE

- With closed eyes, visualize each of your attachments as a stone on your head or back. Feel the weight of all you must carry.

- Now imagine a spirit helper come to assist you. Visualize what this helper looks like. Perhaps an ancestor or relative who has passed over. Or an animal? Or any spirit helper you imagine.

- Now imagine that this spirit helper begins to remove each stone one by one. Feel the lightness as you breathe in and out deeply, releasing the weight. Smile in gratitude to the helper, knowing beyond doubt that you are not alone.

- Write.

- Know that your loved ones will continue as part of you — only the weight will be less as you move through life.

In my workshops, as well as my books, I ask students to do short writing exercises, which are then shared with the group. Once during a five-day workshop at Esalen Institute in Big Sur, California, I presented the exercise to visualize current problems and obstacles as stones piled on the back, and students were then asked to visualize a spirit helper removing the stones one by one. Here is a humorous response from Bill Herr, a wonderful writer from Texas who was taking my workshop again for the fifth year:

This Japanese dude, claiming he was some kind of monk, came up to me and said, "Willy, we're going to use these stones and make a Zen garden. We'll bury them in gravel so they can gestate in the belly of the earth. Every day a monk will come and rake the gravel, and over time the stones will emerge. One of these centuries you will find your burdens released. You just have to be patient."

Home Is Where Our Story Begins

It is thought in some cultures that the soul chooses where it will be born and to whom. What lessons did soul wish you to learn by the path provided? The best guide you have is your own history. But sometimes it helps to create a new perspective on our history. As with all of us, my childhood colors my writing as it does my life perspective. One amazing discovery I have learned is that writing about my own life as honestly as I can has touched the lives of many others in the telling. In the specific resides the universal and not the other way round. No one else can tell your story. Remember that your point of view is unique. And ponder this: "Whom might I help by telling my own story?" Remember, too, that stories create community. Today this community is also global. I often hear from those who are touched by my online courses. People I may never actual meet in person, people from all corners of the globe. One woman from Australia felt I had written the Healing course just for her. A group of Iranian men said they met every week to do *The Way of Story* exercises and now were reading my book for the third time. Through sharing ourselves, we touch others.

EXERCISE

If you were asked to share one experience you had with someone you knew, something experienced as a gift or transmission, what would it be? Close your eyes and see what arises. Which gift will you pass on?

• What is a visual image or metaphor to symbolize this person? This might be an animal, flower, object, a bird, gem, or simply a color.

- Write one page describing the person you have chosen from your own life. Try to focus and bring him or her to life.

- Describe what feelings arise as well as what you learned from this experience.

- Lastly, what attributes of this person do you choose to integrate into your own psyche?

Presence

To be fully centered in the moment is to be present. All of life is a capacity for Presence.

Listen to your dreams, dialogue with them, and integrate their wisdom. Welcome your ancestor, animal, and other spirit guides. Open to the invisible worlds. Allow their guidance and help in removing unwanted baggage and bringing light. Invisible allies are ever there, waiting. All that is needed is to open the portals.

All too often, it is the sense of within and without that interrupts Presence, mere thoughts that separate what is, in truth, One. When we perceive that we are One, there is no problem, no suffering. Thought arises and separates us. It is when we identify with a myriad of thoughts and take them to be real that division occurs. In truth, only silence is real, the Light — not the shadows that come and go.

It is worthwhile taking the time to cultivate Presence. The greatest gift you can give to the moment is Presence. The greatest gift you can offer to another is the same. What if you were able to truly listen to a loved one, to

offer him or her not your advice or opinion — but your
deepest presence?

> *My teacher told me one thing.*
> *Live in the soul.*
> Lalla, female Sufi

Chapter Eight

Discovering Personal Myth: Transcending the Archetype

—◆—

No bird soars too high if he soars with his own wings.
William Blake

How we remember is how we give meaning to a life lived. Often we need look no further for those archetypes or life models than those rich, human imprints from our own childhood. Memory — both personal and collective — remains one of our greatest resources in the journey toward self-knowledge.

Nineteenth-century English novelist Charles Dickens begins his most autobiographical novel, *David Copperfield*, with these lines:

> *Whether I shall turn out to be the hero of my own life, or whether that station will be held by anybody else, these pages must show. To begin my life with the beginning of my life, I record that I was born...*

Science tells us that we genetically inherit both physical and psychological traits, talents, and other tendencies — not only from our parents and grandparents, but also from earlier generations. Freud showed us how childhood experiences exert an influence on adulthood. Jung expanded this to claim that our ancestral and cultural past also exerts an influence on us in our adult lives. Consciously or unconsciously, each of us is living some myth, some archetype imprinted from both the recent or distant past.

Inherited Traits — Both Positive and Negative

My own ancestors came from England, Scotland, Ireland, Wales, and France in the early seventeenth century to Virginia. During the Civil War in America in 1863, while the men were off fighting, the Yankees burned down one branch of my family's barn and threatened my ancestors. To survive, the women and children boarded a covered wagon and made an arduous overland trip to Texas.

Several years ago, my mother passed on to me a diary written by one of these brave women. It was an account of her wagon train trip with nine other Southern families — women and children — from Cedar County, Missouri. I edited Mrs. H. G. Haggard's diary, calling it *A Civil War Memoir (High Roads Folio*, volume 10). Daily challenges included being threatened by the Yankee soldiers who stole their horses and ransacked their belongings, Indians who menaced, rough weather, and the general hardships of broken wagon wheels, illnesses, and lack of food. From these ancestors came a legacy of resilience, boundless courage, and fierce determination. I witnessed these same traits in my maternal grandmother, a direct descendent of pioneer hero Davy Crockett, and am inspired still by the memory of her quiet strength, goodness, and unassuming power.

My ancestor, Mrs. Haggard, writes, "We had been in distress but not discouraged. We knew no such word as fail." Against the greatest of odds, these women and children reached their destination, Texas, where their descendants live to this day. Their spirit lives on and has come to my aid many times in New York, Hollywood, England, France, India, and other far-flung places where I now teach writing workshops.

We all inherit positive traits such as courage, endurance, sense of family, integrity, and so on. Of course, with such positive traits, less desirous ones may also come into play. A tendency toward alcoholism, for instance, runs in this same Southern family. This is not to say that such tendencies are always succumbed to — however, it is useful to recognize them. Negative traits such as alcoholism may take different forms in later generations, such as a craving for sugar or a tendency to become a workaholic.

I am also aware of my Puritan background, which is an association with delayed gratification, focus on work or duty first, exaggerated independence, and self-denial. Being aware of these negative traits has helped me to grow beyond them while at the same time honor those traits that enabled past generations to survive and prosper.

Take some time now to consider your own background. What legacy was passed on to you, both positive and negative?

EXERCISE

- Sit quietly and relax into yourself, perhaps in a deeper way than usual. Use music if that assists.

- Contemplate your ancestral background, where your forebears came from.

- What are their characteristics?

- Write down traits you may have inherited — both positive and negative ones.

- What were your ancestors' beliefs? Their challenges?

- Which ones do you identify with?

To know one's self is the way to freedom. This means becoming aware of the shadow side as well as the light. Remember, there is no light without darkness.

Family Archetypes

There are various modes or styles you may adopt to write your own archetypal story. Choosing one helps to distance you from the story, enabling you to acquire a new vantage point and create a space between you and your story.

Regardless of what negative events are in your own story, remember that we are much more than the sum of our past. Invisible allies are on hand to light the way for re-visioning the past and for healing. There are invaluable lessons waiting for us as we summon our past and those of our forebears. Look first to your roots to find family archetypes to guide you on your journey.

My maternal grandmother grew up on a farm in north Texas near Dallas. One rainy afternoon, she was sharing her past with me, describing how her neighbors shared their crops with one another during the Depression, a challenging time in America. "Oh," I said, "you mean you bartered." "No," she replied firmly. "We gave. We gave, and they gave." With this simple correction, she enabled me to see the past with her eyes. Her perspective was quite different from that of my own generation, for her perspective had more heart. This casual exchange remains a valued legacy long after this wonderful woman passed. Even now, I sometimes imagine my "Gram," her clear blue eyes full of life and understanding, standing behind me. (Twice psychics I have seen have commented on seeing her standing behind me, describing her to a tee!) Positive memories can serve as a powerful ally, for heart memory is stronger even than death.

Despite its power, memory is usually experienced in disjointed fragments. These fragments may make no sense at first yet serve to draw you into a labyrinthine journey, which, if faithfully followed, leads back to a deeper layer of your psyche. An image, a smell, a sound, a phrase of dialogue spoken may precipitate a flood of memories streaming the portals of the mind. You have only to follow. The following exercises may help.

EXERCISE

- Turn now to your own remembrances of things past and choose one amongst your family who influenced your life.

- Describe the person. Be as specific as possible.

- Choose a specific moment with this person and write it down.

- Describe the feelings evoked by this moment in time.

- What value was planted within from knowing this person?

Speak what we feel, not what we ought to say.
William Shakespeare, *King Lear*

EXERCISE

- Choose three family photos. Sit quietly and look carefully at each photo, noting the details. Details reveal much.

- What feelings emerge as you look at the photos?

- Capture the memories and associations that flow through these photos.

EXERCISE

Choose three or all of the following, allowing time to drift and dream. Then when it feels right, write whatever comes.

• Family heroes.

• Ancestor stories.

• What is the image of a good person?

• What is the image of evil?

• Stories of your parents before marriage.

• Stories of yourself as a child. Ones you like? Ones you dislike?

• Suppressed stories of your family.

• Who do you want to be like? Who least so?

• How has your perspective changed when you think or hear these stories?

Memories are not only carried in our conscious and unconscious memory, but also in our senses. For instance, even now, if I smell an apple pie baking anywhere, my grandmother is instantly present. The very smell conjures her up at once.

EXERCISE

- Choose a family photo of one of your parents, grandparents, or another relative.

- Sit quietly in front of the photograph, allowing your mind to drift into memories of things past. Close your eyes.

- Try to remember how this person smelled. Recall his or her touch.

- Then, whether the experience is positive or negative, describe it in words from a feeling perspective.

EXERCISE

Write of a significant event in your life. Choose one or all of the following. Take all the time you need to write.

- Meeting someone who changed your life.

- The birth of someone important to you.

- The moment a respected mentor influenced you.

- The moment you knew what you wanted to be or do.

- A magical moment in nature.

- A special experience while traveling.

- Leaving home for the first time and how you felt then.

- Holidays at home.

- A spiritual experience.

Exploring Past Lives

Apart from ancestors and immediate family who form our personal conscious identity, there may be inherited tendencies from past lives (for those of us aware of such). Exploring probable past lives can expand our sense of who we are and how we came to be so. Have you ever visited a foreign country for the first time and knew beyond doubt that you had lived there before? Or met someone for the first time and yet instantly recognized the person? Similarly, there may be past life tendencies that activate in the proper setting such as a taste or talent for music or performing or dancing or drawing, or a longing for a monastic or spiritual life. Perhaps there lurks within a drive to be powerful or a tendency to avoid power as if some memory from the past obstructs achieving power this time around. It does not matter if you believe in past lives or not. Imagining that one has lived past lives — whether or not one believes — is a marvelous way of accessing other dimensions of the archetypal Self.

EXERCISE

- Imagine or remember a past life that is a positive influence on this life. Write about it.

- Now imagine a past life that has left some unresolved residue in you, which may not be completely positive, or may even be negative, such as a fear or obsession. Write about it.

Survival Archetypes, Patterns, and Personas

Now apart from patterns that we can trace back to past lives, ancestors, and parents, there are some we manage to generate all by ourselves in this life. So let us take some time to consider these as well. Sometimes, we create patterns to help us survive in atmospheres not conducive to growth. Later these same patterns that helped us to survive become our enemies. For instance, if one grows up in a home with domestic violence, to survive one may adapt by learning to be invisible, to not make any waves, or to expect any affection. This can help one survive a challenging childhood yet later may stand in the way of finding love or recognition in work.

The appendix was vital at the time when man ate raw meat. Now we can live without that organ.

I can think of a woman I know who grew up alone and became very independent and strong, with a successful career. That strength carried her through a challenging childhood, one without love. Later on when she met a man who loved her, she could not open to this love. He told her that her problem was that she really didn't need anyone. Surprised at first as she knew this was not true, she began to understand how others saw her. The persona she had so well crafted in order to survive — a persona that walled her in and others out — now obstructed her chance for personal fulfillment.

EXERCISE

- Think of one pattern you have observed about yourself that you feel no longer serves your life plan or goals.

- Write about how it came to be and how it helped you to survive a period in your life.

- Now write a dialogue thanking this trait for helping you to survive and telling it that it is no longer necessary for your life now. Bid it gently adieu.

Sometimes patterns or traits that seem negative have their purpose. For instance, anger may have the power to change history, when channeled positively as anger toward injustice.

EXERCISE

Consider a trait or pattern you or others may feel is negative, and yet, that serves you in some vital way. Write about the plus and minus aspects of this trait or pattern.

Mythic Archetypes

As a way in, let us look at which mythic archetypes we identify with and why. The following exercise might be useful — as well as fun.

EXERCISE

Read the following descriptions of archetypes taken from Greek and Roman gods and goddesses. Choose one or two you identify with and write why.

- Aphrodite (whose Roman name is Venus) is the goddess of love, beauty, pleasure, and procreation. Because of her beauty, other gods feared that jealousy would interrupt the peace among them and lead to war.

- Ares (whose Roman name is Mars) is sometimes viewed as a destructive force. Mars represents military power as a way to secure peace. His affair with Venus is passionate and fiery and gives birth to Mercury, god of communication.

- Hermes (whose Roman name is Mercury) is the messenger who wears winged sandals. Mercury is also a god of trade, thieves, and travel. He has a quick mind and is well travelled.

- Athena (whose Roman name is Minerva) is the goddess of wisdom, courage, inspiration, civilization, law and justice, just warfare, mathematics, strength, strategy, the arts, crafts, and skill. Athena is also a shrewd companion of heroes and is the goddess of heroic endeavor.

- Artemis (whose Roman name is Diana) is the Hellenic goddess of the hunt, wild animals, wilderness, childbirth, virginity, and young girls, bringing and relieving disease in women. She is often depicted as a huntress carrying a bow and arrows.

- Zeus (whose Roman name is Jupiter) is the king of the gods, the god of sky and thunder. As the sky-god, he is a divine witness to oaths. Jupiter's primary sacred animal is the eagle, which holds precedence over other birds.

- If none of these relate, then choose your own archetype. It can be a mythic god, superhero such as Spider-Man, or literary, television, or comic strip character. Just name him or her and expand on how and why this archetype relates to you.

Perhaps more modern depictions speak to you. Here are recent examples from popular television series:

- *The Sopranos*
- *Mad Men*
- *Friday Night Lights*
- *Downton Abbey*
- *Game of Thrones*

All the above television series carry the theme of the fall of the king and the death of the structure that supports the king. Other possible themes are the collapse of the global economy and the depleting ecology of the earth. Think of a more recent television series and choose a character from one you identify with.

> *The gods are in transition, ever-changing.*
> James Hillman

EXERCISE

• Think of a current challenge in your life.

• Now imagine how your archetype would deal with this problem. Write in the first person as if you are Athena or Jupiter or Tony Soprano.

EXERCISE

• Describe your own voice and life perspective in contrast to other voices inherited or learned.

• Describe the voice you wish to nourish within yourself, discarding those that have lived in you uninvited.

Your Personal Myth

Consciously or unconsciously, we are each living our personal myth or archetype. It might be a person or image or subtle guide that guides us from within. There is always some marker looming to which we aspire. Usually, too, the imprints are formed early in life.

The ancient divinities live on through us
and we play out their stories.
David L. Miller, *The New Polytheism*

Which story or myth are you playing out? What myth or fairy tale or icon do you identify with? Snow White? Hansel or Gretel? Marilyn Monroe? Robinson Crusoe? Odysseus? Helen of Troy? The Brady Bunch? Spider-Man?

EXERCISE

• Think of a myth or fairy tale that speaks to you — perhaps one that captured you when you were young — and that serves as a metaphor for your own life's journey. (It can come from anywhere: book, television show, comic strip.)

• First briefly describe the mythic story in a basic storyline.

• Now write about some part of your life and become the archetype you have already described. In other words, you are Snow White, etc. Write in the first person. Choose some part of your own life that connects in some way — real or imagined — to the archetype chosen. You might begin, "I remember myself at age __ when... "

For example, I chose Ariadne, princess of Crete, waiting for her prince to rescue her so she might find her true place. This is an excerpt from what arose for me:

I can remember myself at age seven, sitting outside and watching the long stretch of grassy Texas lawn and an endless driveway dotted with rose bushes, waiting... waiting for someone to come and carry me away to my rightful place. Even as a small child, I knew I did not belong here, that this place was not home. Strange how even when very young, we know where we belong and where we don't. These people were not my people. I was right though it would be many years before I would find my tribe.

The way back to one's deeper Self is not an easy journey yet the only one worth making. To view one's life symbolically and not literally is to discover meaning at every step. It is a never-ending story. Note the key here is to view one's Self and one's journey symbolically and not literally — if only people could view religious texts in the same fashion!

Mythic archetypes are both personal and collective. What happens is not always external. Sometimes an inner image or archetype can prove a more powerful influence on our lives than those we know in real life. Though individual in detail, the archetypal patterns are universal, ever changing, and, unlike dogma or religion, their forms are as varied and as changeless as the sea. Here the multilayered paradox of life and individuals.

The Power of Imagination

Einstein once wrote that imagination is more important than knowledge. We can never underestimate the power of the imagination in healing. A young child escapes a dysfunctional home, climbs a tree, and gazes tranquilly at passing clouds for hours. When imagination comes into play as in transforming the clouds into animals or spirits, this child is being healed of negative imprints suffered at home. Creativity is healing this child. The challenge is to keep the inner child's creative capacity alive as we grow older.

Every child is an artist. The problem is
how to remain an artist once he grows up.
Pablo Picasso

EXERCISE

- If you could be anyone, living or dead, who would you be? And why?

- Go with the first person you think of rather than pondering long. Just take the plunge and write freely, whatever comes. Don't forget to add the why.

Now you are becoming the creative force in your life. How does it feel? Take a moment and feel the power of the creative Self. Where in your body do you feel the energy? Honor that. What we think or imagine is, in fact, our reality — both individually and collectively. This is freedom. Also, there is always choice as to how we will perceive outer reality. What will you choose? Often what you create for yourself is what you love.

If you wish to change your life, change your archetype. Choose the archetype by which to live your life and fulfill your dreams.

Tibetan monks are schooled in the power of visualization. For something to manifest, it must first be visualized. This requires an intensity of focus. Focused journaling can be a tool toward this end. From a blank page, you can create the "something" you wish your life to be. Why not visualize the archetype or blueprint of the authentic life you desire?

Auditions are being held for you to be yourself. Apply within.

EXERCISE

- Create the movie of your life. See the blank movie screen and imagine your story played upon it.

- Genre: romance, action, mystery, or fantasy?

- Setting: place and time?

- Theme?

- Main characters?

- Who would you cast as yourself?

EXERCISE

—◆—

- Describe a day in the life you choose. It can be anywhere on earth. Be specific.

- You can be surrounded by anyone you choose.

- You can be doing anything in the world you wish to do. Be generous to yourself in what you imagine. Write it all down.

> *In our most private and subjective lives*
> *we are not only the passive witnesses*
> *of our age and its sufferers, but also its*
> *makers. We make our epoch.*
>   C. G. Jung

EXERCISE

—◆—

- Now return to the same exercise above and do it again.

- Read it through and ask yourself, "What is different this time?" Write that down as well.

Seeking insight into our moment in history requires narrative content. We enter therapy to seek help in reforming the narrative of our lives. A lack of balance occurs when we lose the narrative thematic thread of our lives. Discover the central thread of your life and hold fast to that.

Early this morning, I walked with a neighbor. He's a gentle guy and a good artist. He shared with me how he is becoming more and more aware of his pattern for choosing neurotic women who use him and give little in return. I asked him, "What is this attraction to neurotic or narcissistic men or women as love partners?" He replied, "I don't know, perhaps a feeling that they need me and I can make a difference in their lives." Here is a man imprisoned by an archetype: the maiden waiting to be rescued. Unconsciously, he is searching for Snow White, Cinderella, or Rapunzel. So when he finds someone manifesting this archetype, he is inevitably captured, becoming himself a prisoner to the archetype. This may be totally unconscious but nonetheless remains a powerful force in his life.

Becoming aware of the archetype that drives us helps us to discover who we are and what we truly want. Each of us seeks a way home to meaning, and from meaning, purpose.

All we have are symbols, metaphors.
Robert Bella

And yet it is the symbol or archetype that is the door to self-understanding, as well as how the world is perceived and revealed to us. Remember — either consciously or unconsciously — we are living our own metaphors.

There is nothing in the Universe
That you are not
Everything you want, look for it
Within yourself. You are that.

Rumi

Chapter Nine

Overcoming Trauma: Beyond Traditional Psychology

In a dark time, the eye begins to see.
Theodore Roethke

Undergoing trauma can set in motion a destructive fragmentation, splitting us off from ourselves. What once was real can become empty form. Little by little, even if we never consciously think of the past, the trauma or grief lives on in us — both mentally and bodily — unacknowledged yet sometimes as active as a diseased cell. Perhaps a feeling of numbness overtakes us. We may find ourselves going through the motions of living, wondering why it is we feel nothing. We begin to lose touch with the sacredness of life. It is even possible to be unaware that we are drifting slowly into a black hole.

In the Introduction, I mentioned briefly the young woman who was a participant in my *Heal Yourself with Writing* seminar, a three-day workshop at the Esalen Institute in Big Sur, California. At thirty-five, she had already made her money in Silicon Valley. As the workshop progressed, a deep sadness emanated from her. We explored the participants' own stories in focused journaling exercises. Some of the participants disclosed powerful, painful moments from their lives, yet she did not. I felt her sadness, but beyond safe, superficial details, I never really heard her share her story though she did all the writing exercises. Perhaps the workshop didn't quite reach her or her time to heal hadn't quite arrived. However, a week later she sent me an email out of the blue, telling me that the three days of focused journaling had done what years of therapy had not. It allowed her to return to herself, to reintegrate with the person she had been as a young teen — before the sexual trauma. At the age of fifteen she had been sexually assaulted by her own brother and one of his friends. After that trauma, she felt forever separated from her body. This profound disassociation may have allowed her to survive, even thrive in the world. But she had longed to return to herself, to reintegrate and become whole. In those three short days, she had found the road home. She shared with me that our days together had allowed her to step back and see her whole life from a different perspective, releasing the role of powerless victim carried all these years.

How did such a transformation occur in so short a period of time? In part, she was ready to heal the split within, but did not know how. Her openness gave her the courage to explore stories about herself that she had not been willing to face before — no matter where such stories might lead. It is also important to add that she wrote the focused journaling exercises in such a way as to create a distance between the past trauma and herself today, aiding her to release their hold. Though imprinted by the past, we are not our past. Each moment of every day offers an opportunity to begin anew.

You must carry chaos inside you to give
birth to a dancing star.
Friedrich Nietzsche

Toward the end of *Harry Potter and the Chamber of Secrets*, Harry Potter has been wounded by the evil snake's poison in the underground chamber. He believes it is fatal until a red phoenix appears and bends over him. Then a tear from the phoenix falls upon the wound, healing him. The young girl Harry has saved is concerned and Harry tells her, "It's all right. It's over. It's just a memory. The phoenix has healing powers."

"It's just a memory" is an invaluable insight. And memory is only thought. And yet, past memories — especially negative ones — can dominate the present and affect the future. In mythology, the phoenix is believed dead yet rises from the ashes to begin a new life. What matters is not only what occurred but how you remember past trauma, and to create a shift wherein you can stand and from which you can remember. In witnessing from a separate perspective, you create a new relationship with what has happened in the past. In this space created between you and the event, healing can occur. This space can offer new meaning as well as a new freedom from the past.

The world does not change. You change. Perspective is all.

EXERCISE

• Write about a lie you were told.

• How did it make you feel at that time?

• What gives it power over you now?

> *I shall allow no man to belittle my*
> *soul by making me hate him.*
> Booker T. Washington

Here's a Zen story to illustrate perception and illusion given us by editor Paul Reps in his wonderful collection, *Zen Flesh, Zen Bones.*

The Zen master Hakuin was praised by one and all as one living a pure life. A beautiful Japanese girl whose parents owned a food store lived near him. One day her parents discovered she was with child. At first, the girl refused to name the father, but after much pressure, she at last named Hakuin. In great anger, the parents marched over to the Zen master, and Hakuin responded by saying, "Is it so?"

After the child was born, it was brought to Hakuin. Now, his reputation lost, he did not seem troubled, and took very good care of the child. A year later the child's mother could stand it no longer and told her parents the truth: that the real father was a young man who worked in the fish market. The parents rushed to Hakuin to beg his forgiveness and to get the child back again. Hakuin simply gave the child back to them, saying, "Is it so?"

What changed? Nothing changed except the perspective. Bad things will happen to us as well as good and wonderful things. Control is often a mechanism of survival.

Yet sometimes we have no control over outer events in our lives or those of our loved ones. What we do have control over is how we perceive and remember. Here creativity can play a powerful role, transforming trauma into transformational growth and meaning.

> *I love the dark hours of my being*
> *In which my senses drop into the deep.*
> *I have found in them, as in old letters,*
> *My private life that is already lived through,*
> *And become wide and powerful now, like legends.*
> *Then I know that there is room in me*
> *For a second huge and timeless life.*
> Rainer Maria Rilke

To embrace a new huge and timeless life, it may be necessary to heal what has gone before.

In the fourth century BC, people would come to sleep at the Temple of Asclepius at Epidaurus, believing that during the dark night, healing would come to them in their dreams. They had only to ask. Even today, dreams possess a healing power.

EXERCISE

- Before sleep, close your eyes, breathing deeply from the soul.

- Simply ask for healing and guidance, being as specific as possible. Trust the process and try not to expect instant results.

- Note whatever words or images arise.

- Meditate on them the next day.

In antiquity, illness was understood as an estrangement from God, while healing was considered to be a reconnection to the transcendent. These were times when humanity was inextricably connected to the divine. However, with the development of our personal and collective psyche, the immediacy of this relationship has been lost. A bridge to the transpersonal is required, helping us to discover a deeply meaningful approach to spirit that allows us to align with our own destiny. Creativity can be such a bridge, a therapeutic approach to healing trauma and grief, making it possible to heal the split in order to find balance and become whole.

Simply relating a past trauma or grief is not enough, and may even retraumatize the body and mind, securing negative patterns and cementing a memory of the event that is based on victimhood. A shift in perspective is what is needed. Using creative tools — such as writing — to shift perspective away from a victim mentality can empower us to self-heal.

EXERCISE

- Discover your own inner compass for feeling good. Visualize a pleasant memory from the past, one that makes you feel safe and happy. Practice returning to this memory in detail.

- Develop the inner muscles to change your thoughts in moments. Deep breathing often helps to shift away from a challenging moment and gather our force from within.

- Recalibrate your perspective. After practicing the first two steps already mentioned, there is time to shift how you perceive what is happening.

- Then you will be in a stronger position to respond and to act.

What we achieve inwardly will change
outer reality.
Plutarch

Of course, some healing needs are more subtle and don't issue from traumatic experiences. A few examples might be trying to reconcile spirituality with money, experiencing a split between the wish to support one's family versus the desire to follow one's dreams. The more aware we become of these needs, the more equipped we are to realize our dreams and live fully in each moment of our lives.

EXERCISE

- Choose a need of yours that, though not large or traumatic, in some way interrupts the flow of your life. Look at it squarely.

- Describe it.

- Now write about it from the perspective of a wise guide. Visualize metaphors or characters for each point of view.

- Perhaps you might try a dialogue between this personal need and a deeper, wiser guide within.

EXERCISE

In this exercise, stay in tune with how you are feeling. If it feels too much at any time, just stop and return to it later. Only you can judge what is right for you and when, so please continue at your own pace and readiness.

- Write, in a few words, a trauma that affected your own life. It might be something done to you or a grief that took possession of you, making it difficult to move on.

- Now, from a new perspective of a hero or heroine undergoing a trial, in a few words, write the same story of the grief or trauma. A hero is never daunted, seeing only the challenge ahead, and focusing on how to overcome it, in some way. Write in the first person.

• This time, write from the soul's point of view, and include the lesson or insight gained because of what happened. What was needed as seen from the longer view of the soul's continuous journey — what it required for soul's growth. The soul can seem ruthless, at times, for it focuses on the long view and its own evolution. A Tibetan monk, only a young boy, had witnessed horrible acts of violence upon his fellow monks by the Chinese at his monastery in Lhasa. When a social worker asked him what he was feeling, his reply was, "The poor Chinese. What bad karma they are creating for themselves."

• Try to adopt this point of view while completing the final and the most challenging part of this exercise. You will be again writing about the trauma or cause of grief that occurred in the past, only this time, write entirely from the point of view of the one you believe is to blame for what happened. Write in the first person.

> *The world into which we are born is*
> *brutal and cruel, and at the same time,*
> *of divine beauty.*
>   C. G. Jung

The Missing Piece

Sometimes we may feel that there are missing pieces in our lives, something not given which leaves a hole in our psyches. Did it ever occur to you that you have the power to replace that missing piece? For instance, if you lacked being properly mothered, it is possible later to become that good mother to yourself. In this manner, we are able to reclaim a life denied to us.

As a child, the only books in my home were the *King James Bible* and a set of encyclopedias called *The Book of Knowledge*, which I devoured from A to Z. No one read children's books to me, and I was not taken to a public library until the age of twelve. Years passed. Then, at twenty-one, I married and a year later gave birth to a son. As he grew, I began buying children's books, and reading them to my son. It was an enriching experience as we together discovered the stories for the first time. Crying at the end of *Charlotte's Web*, moved speechless when the fox was tamed (i.e., loved) by the Little Prince. Later on, this became a family ritual as my son and I took turns reading aloud to each other the novels of Charles Dickens and other authors. Through reading to my son, I recovered that missing piece from childhood. Nothing is lost to us, if we remain open to receive. Never forget that you have the power to give to yourself that missing piece.

EXERCISE

— ◆ —

• Consider for a moment a missing piece from your childhood. Close your eyes and feel the hole within.

• Describe that hole. What color is it? What shape?

• Now imagine a situation in real or imagined life where you are being given that missing piece.

• Remember, too, that sometimes in order to receive what we need, we must first give it to someone else. In the process of giving, it comes back to us. Write of such an example from your own life.

Taking Responsibility for One's Life

Though many of us have endured challenging times and even terrible events in our lives, at some point we have to say, "Enough." It is time to take responsibility for what is and will be my life. Just say "no" to negative patterns that no longer serve. Create a daily habit of positive thoughts and feelings. Regardless of what is going on with families or friends or work, there is a beautiful sunrise waiting for you to view. A robin will sing for all who care to listen. And there is always someone there to listen to our song, if we take proper care in how we put it out there.

Even after taking responsibility for our lives, memories of past grief and traumas may still arise. See them as uninvited guests arriving on your doorstep. Greet them with compassion but with firmness. Tell them there is no room for them in your house now.

Pain is inevitable. Suffering is optional.
Dalai Lama

When you tire of suffering, it is time to begin the spiritual work. Suffering arises when we resist. Once we accept what is, then suffering loses its force. A flowing river moves boulders.

Letting Go of What No Longer Serves

One does not become enlightened by imagining figures of light, but by making the darkness conscious.
C. G. Jung

Sometimes unconsciously we just won't let go of what no longer serves. Emotionally we feel old destructive patterns serve us in some way. They may constitute how we see ourselves and the world around us. Even patterns or perspectives that no longer serve are familiar while change can be frightening.

EXERCISE

• Think of one habit inherited from a parent that no longer serves and that you are ready to release.

Close your eyes, and with compassion and without judgment, thank this habit or trait for staying close so many years and helping you to get this far. Tell it you are ready to bid it good-bye. Visualize seeing it leave.

- Take three deep breaths in gratitude.

- Now, visualize an affirmation that you choose to adopt into your life. It may be the opposite of the trait released. Write it down. Write it down two more times.

- Now close your eyes and repeat it to yourself as you smile.

> *All true things must change,*
> *and only that which changes remains true.*
> C. G. Jung

EXERCISE

- Think of one pattern you have observed about yourself that you feel no longer serves your life plan or goals.

- Perhaps write about how it came to be and how it helped you to survive a period in your life.

- Now write a dialogue thanking this trait for helping you to survive and telling it that it is no longer necessary for your life now.

In this process of letting go of conditioned patterns, we must be alert not to throw out the baby with the bathwater, so to speak. Sometimes patterns or traits that seem negative have their purpose. For instance, personal suffering can give birth to compassion for others.

EXERCISE

- Consider a trait you or others may feel is negative even though it may serve in some vital way.

- Write about the plus and minus aspects of this trait or pattern.

Once you identify the negative traits and patterns and their origin, it is necessary to stay alert to their voices and not heed them. Know that they are not your own voice. The more you listen to and strengthen your own authentic voice, the more the lesser ones will recede as uninvited guests from your home.

EXERCISE

- Describe your own voice and life perspective in contrast to other voices inherited or learned.

- Describe the voice you wish to nourish within yourself, discarding those that have lived in you, uninvited.

Often in the midst of daily survival, we forget one very important and sometimes life-changing factor: there is always choice. In other words, to choose how we view what is happening to us. In this power of choice, lies power.

EXERCISE

- Become very still. Take three slow breaths, focusing on the breathing in and out. Feel your body breathing.

- Now visualize your thoughts rising and leaving, as guests in your house. It is not that negative thoughts will go away entirely — only lose their power over us in time.

- Remember that you are the space wherein life happens.

> *We don't receive wisdom; we must discover it for ourselves after a journey that no one can take for us, or spare us.*
> Marcel Proust

However, life growth is not only about letting go of what no longer serves. It may also include retrieving what has been lost.

EXERCISE

- Write about what you regret having let go of in your life in the past.

- Now add what stops you from welcoming it back into your life now.

> *I am the dream you are dreaming.*
> *When you want to awaken, I am waiting.*
> Rainer Maria Rilke

When others who depend on you ask for more and more, always keep yourself on that list of who you must help and care for. Ultimately, the best way to change anyone is by living your own truth.

> *In the world of knowledge,*
> *Every day something new is added.*
> *In pursuit of the Tao,*
> *Every day something is let go.*
> Lao Tzu

The Alchemy of Compassion

The word compassion means "shared sorrow." Sometimes when we can expand our specific sorrow or wound to embrace all others who have suffered a similar wrong or injury, it can alleviate our own.

EXERCISE

—◆—

- Close your eyes and let arise in your mind any particular suffering or sorrow you experience or have experienced. Hold the vision of this for a moment. Breathe into it. If it concerns a part of your body, breathe into that part.

- Now envision a violet light as you inhale and draw to your body this sorrow. Let it fill your body. Envision whatever form or color it may take. Hold this for a moment.

- Now allow this embodied suffering to expand in a spirit of compassion embracing all souls who have suffered as you have. Watch the light widen expanding outward, and with it see your suffering now transformed into the bright white light of compassion for all.

- Now breathe easily in and out, transmuting the energy of pain and sorrow into that of love and compassion for all who have suffered in this world.

Sometimes unlearning is the most important learning. Change can be a frightening proposition. Often it seems easier to cling to familiar patterns rather than let go of them and trust the inner process of soul evolution. Often what we resist, that is, changing and growing, is what is most needed. And when we resist too long, some outer crisis may occur to force us to see.

The Chinese ideogram for the word *crisis* also means "opportunity." Without such moments in history or in our singular lives, there is no discovery, no evolution.

EXERCISE

- List three things about yourself that you sometimes find it difficult to accept.

- List three things about yourself that you are willing to change.

- Engage an inner dialogue with that part of yourself and embrace the courage needed to let go and move on.

Once you have identified the negative traits and patterns and their origin, it is necessary to stay alert to their voices and not heed them. Know that they are not your own voice. The more you listen to and strengthen your own authentic voice, the more the lesser ones will recede.

Listen. Make a way for yourself inside yourself.
Rumi

EXERCISE

———◆———

• Describe your own voice and life perspective in contrast to other voices inherited or learned.

• Describe the voice you wish to nourish within yourself, discarding those that have lived in you, uninvited. Write in the first person.

Beyond Trauma

There is no need for despair, regardless of how many years we have lived in this manner, for each and every moment is an opportunity for rebirth. This is the essence of the creative process, one example being focused journaling. To become a co-creator of your life requires only that you find the courage to be in touch with what is happening day by day, moment by moment. Black holes when faced squarely and aided by creativity and courage can be transformed into light, giving birth to a new and vital life full of meaning and purpose. For this, however, courage is needed.

In the harsh brightness of the modern world, we have grown unaccustomed to darkness, sometimes even fearing it. For nine months we rested contentedly in our mother's womb in darkness, yet now blinded by industrialized lights, we have forgotten how to find our way home. Life arises from and returns to darkness; such is the cycle of life. In the same manner, from the dark periods of life, a new consciousness may arise. The dark cycles are sometimes necessary for transitioning us from one place to another. A metaphorical death symbolizes the end of one life in order for a new life to be. Without the death of stars, there would be no earth or other planets. The process of creation is one of chaos, breakdown, and destruction which, in turn, fuels new beginnings. In all creation myths, there exists a time of darkness before the dawn of the new world.

Don't forget that just when the caterpillar thinks the world has ended, it becomes a butterfly.

> *In the middle of the journey of our life*
> *I found myself in a dark wood,*
> *For I had lost the right path.*
> *And so we came forth,*
> *and once again beheld the stars.*
>   Dante, *Inferno*

Chapter Ten

Creating Space and Time for Inner Growth

The voyage of discovery is not in seeking new landscapes, but in having new eyes.
Marcel Proust

Today ours is a culture of distraction with little space left in between for contemplation. Our culture focuses on progress, achievement, and ascent — sometimes forgetting that the sun itself must also descend. The descent of the sun parallels the unconscious depth that is discovered as we descend within. Since we are not machines, space and time are needed for this essential life process.

Sometimes we need unscheduled time in our lives, solitude to explore within. This helps to balance the busy daily external lives we all live.

I think back with gratitude to the lazy, drifting hours of a Texas childhood when I, an only child, was simply left alone to lay back on the grass and watch passing clouds. I attribute these hours to the development of imagination which later earned my living in New York and Hollywood. Cloud-gazing is time well spent. Today, with the best of intentions, small, preschool children are scheduled tightly with classes of all kinds. How important it is to allow the young unscheduled, non-competitive, non-goal-oriented to explore within and to create without! Actually, this is true at any age. When Virginia Woolf spoke of the need for women writers to have "a room of one's own," I believe she meant this.

I like people. I enjoy being with friends, even going to an occasional party. And yet, I've noticed that when down time is not firmly scheduled, something goes awry, and the balance shifts. There is a physical and psychic need for solitude. Sometimes it is vital to be left alone. This is a time when we honor and support a relationship to the Self. From this first primal relationship, all other relationships come.

Nonetheless, sometimes restlessness or impatience may arise when you are alone. Resist sometimes the temptation to turn on the television or call someone just to chat. When impatience or restlessness is felt during alone times, try this exercise.

EXERCISE

- Sit in a beautiful place, if possible, in a garden or by a window with a view of something soothing.

- Then close your eyes and simply listen. At first hear the external sounds, whether a bird or passing cars. Then allow yourself to sink deeper within and listen to your own thoughts. At first, it may be surface thoughts ("I must pick up butter at the store" or some such).

- Stay focused and sink deeper still. At some point, you will feel a settling into a deeper place within. Then listen to any guidance which Self may offer. This takes little time and is time well spent.

- You might keep a journal nearby to record what arises from the deeper you.

> *It does not matter how slowly you go*
> *As long as you do not stop.*
> Confucius

EXERCISE

- Visualize your house.

- Now imagine discovering a room never before seen. In fact, you didn't even know this room existed until now.

- Enter this room. Describe it.

- Now describe how it feels to be in this new room, this new space.

The Pace of Life

There is more to life than increasing its speed.
Mohandas K. Gandhi

As I've mentioned, in my twenties and thirties, I lived in Manhattan, worked in the theatre as an actress then playwright and taught for several years at The New

School University. Becoming a single parent, I also raised a son. (Though, I might also say that he raised me.) Life in New York was fast paced and my schedule always full. It has of late occurred to me that even now — decades later — I am still over-scheduling myself, travelling all the time to teach globally, and basically still living a New York fast-paced life. At least this was so until quite recently. What happened to change this?

Jung once said that if we don't listen to the inner voice telling us to make a change, something will manifest to get our attention. Well, I didn't listen to that little voice that said, "Time to slow down." I felt that I could still function as I did when twenty-eight. I scheduled many teaching gigs back to back, and in England and France alone, I had slept in thirteen beds in three weeks. Returning to the States, I taught at three places in and near New York before flying home to California. On the flight home from JFK Airport, exhausted, I contracted the swine flu virus, which later hit my inner ear giving me a challenging case of vertigo for eighteen months. Well, the message was clear: slow down. Funny thing about having vertigo is that there is absolutely no choice. You have to slow down due to the severe dizziness. Illness is a humbling experience. You confront vulnerability and realize that health is not something to take for granted. It was challenging both physically and emotionally. And yet, what was at first debilitating, i.e., vertigo, later became a sacred messenger. I was made to respect the body and its limitations at certain times in life. A shift long overdue came to light, and at long last, I listened.

Of course, it is always best to stay tuned and listen to the inner voice before an accident or disease strikes. However, some of us are a bit stubborn and may require an extra nudge. In any case, a shift in perspective occurred.

In the rush of today's world, it is natural to be swept up in an unnatural pace and later to feel overwhelmed. At such times, before illness or accidents force us, it is wise to create time and space to replenish the well and restore balance.

Replenishing the Well

I always wonder why birds stay in the same place when they can fly anywhere on the earth. Then I ask myself the same question.
Harun Yahya

Sometimes it is crucial to simply stay in one place and turn inward — at least for a time, allowing ourselves the opportunity to discover untapped resources within. Another wonderful thing about allowing uninterrupted time and space for the Self is the luxury of allowing a slower process of deciding without having to force a decision. Even now, I make sure I sleep on it before making any important decision.

Here is a personal example. Characteristically, once I commit to something, I generally follow through. After committing to present a keynote talk in London and teach in New York this fall, I recently awoke with a clear intuitive message to cancel both engagements —

something I rarely, if ever, do. However, I knew I needed to stay put to replenish myself and to complete this book. As there was ample time for them to replace me, I called and cancelled. As soon as I did as my inner voice instructed, I felt a warm glow of having served the Self. Delighted that I have more time home than usual, I feel liberated and inspired to write more — as well as to exercise more!

Don't let yesterday use up too much of today.
Cherokee Indian Proverb

EXERCISE

Imagine you are travelling to a desert isle. What would you take with you? Why this choice?

- One piece of music.

- One book.

- One person.

- One pet.

EXERCISE

- Without undue thinking, write down five favorite words.

- Now write whatever associations arise from each word.

Being Centered, Seeing Clear

To see a world in a grain of sand
And a heaven in a wild flower,
Hold infinity in the palm of your hand
And eternity in an hour.
   William Blake

Let's do another solitary walk while searching for a new metaphor.

EXERCISE

• Take a solitary walk where there is beautiful nature.

• Search for a metaphor to symbolize something you feel strongly about. It might be a characteristic such as a dying plant symbolizing that we all will die, or a bird or animal that reminds you of a teacher you once had. Perhaps a hen that kept finding fault, pecking away at the student's self-esteem. Or a late-blooming plant symbolizing how life renews itself.

• Explore in writing whatever story or associations arise from the metaphor.

• What feeling does this metaphor and these associations evoke in you?

Along with cloud-gazing and seeing, inner listening is also important. When was the last time you truly listened to what was happening within you?

> *The old voice of the ocean,*
> *the bird-chatter of little rivers.*
> *From different throats intone one language.*
> *So I believe if we were strong enough*
> *to listen without Divisions of desire and terror*
> *To the storm of the sick nations,*
> *the rage of the hunger-smitten cities.*
> *Those voices also would be found...*
> Robinson Jeffers, *Natural Music*

EXERCISE

- Play some favorite, soothing music.

- Sit in a comfortable place or lie down.

- Close your eyes, tuning out the outer world.

- Simply turn within and listen.

- Later write whatever associations arise.

EXERCISE

- Take a leisurely trip to your local library and choose books that will nourish your soul. Or browse Amazon or your Kindle and do the same.

• During this time of creating space and time for inner growth, purchase a handsome journal and cultivate a practice of writing something in it daily as a way of dialoguing with your deeper Self.

Years ago during my Fulbright research year in India, I took my teenage son out of school so that he could come along on this adventure. There were two conditions that he agreed to: doing his lesson plans so that he would not miss a year of school and keeping a journal. Later he told me that his journal was his best friend.

> *If there's a book you really want to read*
> *but it hasn't been written yet, then you*
> *must write it.*
> Toni Morrison

Life Is Relationship

People only see what they are prepared to see.
Ralph Waldo Emerson

Living is relationship — both with your Self and others. A balanced life requires both. As was said earlier, the most important relationship is with your Self. Yet other relationships matter as well, and will thrive best when we are at one with ourselves.

In his excellent book, *The Way of Transformation: Daily Life as Spiritual Practice,* Austrian philosopher

Karlfried Graf Durckheim states that man has basically three needs in life in order to find fulfillment:

- basic survival of food and shelter

- a sense of meaning and purpose

- dialogue

The first two were easy to comprehend, but it took me some years before I fully understood what Durckheim meant by "dialogue." I feel Durckheim is referring here to a need to meaningfully connect to another, to mirror our deeper self with another human being. So the need for communication is essential. We do not live in a vacuum unless it's one of our own making. The very need to communicate arises from inherently knowing or sensing that we are connected with all that surrounds us — nature, animals, others.

> *We are but one thread within it.*
> *Whatever we do to the web,*
> *We do to ourselves.*
> *All things are bound together.*
> *All things connect.*
>   Chief Seattle, 1855

To live from a unified soul is a powerful thing. John Stuart Bell, the Irish physicist, speaks of what is now called Bell's Theorem: that any two atoms, once having encountered the other, will forever be connected and influence the other, regardless of their distance from each other. Beyond cause and effect is where the potential of life is.

Discovery has meaning only in relationship. And communication is the expression of this relatedness. The very root of the word, *communication*, is the same as *communion* or an act of sharing. However, for true communication to be, we must first create a healthy communication with our deeper Self. If we project division outwardly as an expression of our own shadow, there can be no true relatedness or communication. First we must experience oneness within.

Looking Outward

It is important to create a balance of cultivating awareness of the outer world as well as that of the inner landscape of soul. The more you are tuned into the inner Self, the more aware you will be of what is perceived without. Here is an exercise to strengthen outer awareness.

EXERCISE

Take another solitary walk in some beautiful area. This time search for a metaphor for what you are experiencing within or as a symbol for some theme you have been contemplating. For instance, once I saw a large rock some yards from shore on Orcas Island, Washington. It was bare rock and yet at the top of the boulder sprouted a flower. I interpreted it as a metaphor for the resiliency and persistence of life.

- Search for a metaphor while walking and gazing.
- What ties you to this metaphor at this particular moment?

Looking Again at What Is Familiar

People alter so much that there is something new to be observed in them forever.
Jane Austen

Who hasn't had the experience of not noticing some vital change in a loved one we see daily? Perhaps it is only new clothes or a new hairstyle or something more, like a change in mood caused by depression or a juicy secret. Just for a week, commit to taking notice of what is familiar and then expressing it to a loved one or friend.

EXERCISE

Describe a time when you neglected to notice some change in a loved one until he or she, or someone else, called it to your attention later.

Listening to Your Inner Voice

Space and silence are needed in order to listen to our deeper selves, our souls that often manifest as intuition. Here is a personal story that illustrates this.

Rajeshwar Dayal was a wonderful man and a fine friend. He worked with Dag Hammarskjöld at the

United Nations, was ambassador from India to France, and later served as Foreign Minister in Indira Gandhi's cabinet. Years later, Rajeshwar mailed me a copy of his autobiography, *A Life of Our Times* (Orient Longman, 1998) which characteristically was about everyone around him more than himself. Usually I would read the whole book before replying to a writer friend, but after reading only twenty pages, some intuition urged me not to wait to reply. So I wrote a letter admiring his book and received a prompt and pleased response. Later I was told that my friend passed a day or two after he replied to my letter. His last words to his wife were:

I go, you go, everything goes. Only the Truth remains.

Listen to your inner voice — even if logically it makes no sense — it's never wrong. If I had waited to write to him, it would have been too late. So perhaps it is important to stop our scurrying, and now and then, feel the essence of the moment. After all, this is all we really have.

During my last annual retreat in south India, I chose the luxury of deep leisure. A favorite pastime was sitting on the veranda, watching the wonderful variety of birds there, and simply staring into space in utter stillness.

There is nothing to do, nowhere to go, no one to be. Perhaps this is the real work of life, the soul's work of surrendering to the Self.

Find What You Love and Follow

Often when I am teaching workshops or speaking at conferences, I am asked how I find the discipline to write. I often reply with this true story.

Many years ago, when I arrived in New York City, a young and fledging actress, I met the writer, Gerald Sykes, and his artist wife, Buffy Johnson. One afternoon, Buffy invited me to her studio. I was amazed at her oil paintings, similar to those of Georgia O'Keeffe — only more intricate. One painting would take months to complete. I remarked on her great discipline to do such work. Still painting, she remarked, "Don't you know? Discipline is love." Buffy Johnson is gone now but not the lesson she taught me. Her splendid paintings may be found in the Metropolitan Museum of Art in New York City. Hers was a labor of love — not discipline. And yet, I have never discovered a better definition of discipline than hers.

> *The more you are motivated by love,*
> *the more fearless and free your action will be.*
>   Dalai Lama

EXERCISE

———◆———

- Sit in stillness as though you have all the time in the world.

- Then ask yourself, "What is it I love?" "What do I wish to do more than anything else because I love doing it?"

- Listen carefully to what arises and write it down.

EXERCISE

———◆———

How to transform your life as it is today?

- Describe a daily practice such as meditating, writing, painting, walking.

- Describe a potential project that excites you. Be as specific as possible.

- Describe activities with loved ones you would like to do.

Coming Home

In the course of our journeys both inner and outer, we find more than once the distinct feeling that we have come home. My first trip to India was one such experience.

The first time I acted in a play felt like coming home. Meeting a kindred spirit that grew into a deep friendship is yet another example of coming home.

EXERCISE

—————

- Make a list of moments in your life that were a "coming home" experience.

- Describe one, including how it felt.

You have explored many rich and profound territories of your own experience through the exercises offered in this book. Perhaps you might now gather together your writings into a compilation. You may want to bind the pages together as a manuscript, or place them between the covers of a beautiful sheath, as was done in ages past. This symbolic book will pay tribute to the journey of your Self through writing. It will be a book without end, ever expanding throughout the moments, days, and years of your life.

Coming home is the longest journey and the most important. I travel the world and seldom rest from my quest. After years of wandering, I stop, become quite still, and turn within... only to realize that home has been there all along, for home is the centered Self. Once you are at home within, you are at home anywhere and everywhere.

Take rest in life. Open the portals of your heart and truly listen to the guidance within. Something is lovingly calling you home to the essence of your being.

How could the soul not take flight
When from the glorious Presence
A soft call flows sweet as honey,
And whispers, "Rise up now, come away."
…How could the hawk not fly away,
Back, back, to the wrist of the king
As soon as he hears the drum
The king's baton hits again and again,
Drumming out the signal of return?
How could the Sufi not start to dance,
Turning on himself, like the atom in the sun of eternity,
So he can leap free of this dying world?
Fly away, fly away, bird, to your native home.
You have leaped free of the cage,
Your wings are flung back in the wind of God.
Leave behind the stagnant and marshy waters,
Hurry, hurry, hurry, O bird, to the source of life!

Rumi (translated by Andrew Harvey)

Chapter Eleven

Looking Back,
Growing Forward

---

*It is our inward journey that leads us
through time — forward or back, seldom
in a straight line, most often spiraling...
As we discover, we remember; remembering,
we discover.*
  Eudora Welty

I believe in story, its power to heal, to transform, and to offer the gift of beginning again. There is a magic in riding a narrative to its end — a magic that allows us to create a new ending altogether. This magic lets us go beyond the rehashing and minute analyzing of some more limited therapies, and sometimes allows us to re-vision our lives.

Change is the very movement of life. It can also be the factor we most resist. To resist change is to resist life itself. When we undergo a crisis or major turning point, it is not uncommon to experience an identity crisis as well. At these times, when we are no longer sure of what we are, we may turn back to a time when we did know. It is natural to look back in order to be in touch with a time when we knew who we were and what our purpose was.

Some years back, when I was writing for the popular television series, *Touched by an Angel*, I created a story, loosely based on my childhood, about a little girl who heard angel voices. Those around her taunted her. One angel observing this on the school playground asked, "Why is it since human beings are born knowing who they are, why is it they forget?" Then the older angel (played by Della Reese) replies, "They call it education." Once we knew who we are. This forgotten, we spend our lives retracing our steps back home.

Sometimes this may extend to physically retracing our steps back to wherever home was or a place where we first discovered our identity and purpose. In this way, the past can serve us. However, it is best to take the journey as a symbolic individual pilgrimage rather than a literal regression to the past. For example, one cannot recapture lost youth, solely by marrying a younger spouse. Life is a journey — not a destination. Each moment of each day is an eternity.

> *Fundamental insights gained from our*
> *own personal perceptions, feelings, and*
> *thoughts are likely to be of more value to*
> *us than insights gained in any other way.*
> Arthur Schopenhauer

The Embodied Soul

Kierkegaard once said that we understand our lives backward, but must live them forward. However, to truly move forward, we must be in touch with our bodies as well as our hearts and minds. Eugene T. Gendlin, in his groundbreaking book, *Focusing*, speaks of the *felt sense* of experience. When there is tension in the body, it is a clue to what is stuck. Trauma is about being stuck. Sometimes a holding pattern becomes habitual, causing tension on the physical level. Physical symptoms are the body's way of communicating. Learn to listen to your body. Without judging, just be aware of your body. Listen to it. Be aware of physical shifts while doing these exercises. The body often knows before the conscious mind. Sensation can be a doorway to freedom. Feel the loosening as you let go of the past. Remember that to remain stuck is to believe that the past is more powerful than the present. It isn't.

> *Of all the creatures of Earth, only human beings*
> *can change their pattern. Man alone is the*
> *architect of his destiny. The greatest revolution*
> *in our generation is that human beings, by*
> *changing the inner attitudes of their minds,*
> *can change the outer aspects of their lives.*
>   William James

Be aware of which thoughts are remnants of your past. Memories, too, are only thoughts. Thoughts can be changed. *Remember it is not what happens that is important, it is your reaction and attitude to what happens.* Be creative. Use happy memories to water the small seed of becoming whole.

Sometimes you may forget to listen to your body in the daily rush of life. It, too, has a voice. To be whole, it is necessary to integrate all the parts of yourself. Soul is embodied so it is important to listen not only to the mind or inner Self, but also to the body.

Be aware of which part of your body is speaking. In the next exercise, give that specific body part a voice.

EXERCISE

Often there is one area of our physical being that is rather like Achilles' heel, the vulnerable part. This is the place where we are sometimes troubled.

- Pick one part of your body. First write about it from your own perspective.

- Next write about that part of your body from *its* point of view.

- Lastly, write a dialogue between the part of the body and yourself. Try to make the other understand what memories are held, and how it and you feel today.

EXERCISE

- Take three slow breaths.

- Be aware, watch breathing in and out. Focus. Feel your body breathing.

- Now visualize yourself as a lotus floating on top of a lovely pond, the roots firmly in the mud, the flower opening to the sky.

- Let go. Allow yourself to float.

- Write what arises from this centered place.

The Gift of Empathy

Leo Tolstoy initially planned to write a novel condemning adultery. Then unintentionally, he fell in love with his own creation, Anna Karenina, and more than a century later, our love for this complex fictional woman only continues to grow. Empathy can transform judgment into love. Similarly, it is possible, with acquired distance and imagination, to feel empathy for those we feel have harmed us or harmed those we love. Healing, when aided by creativity, can be experienced as an act of compassion for the past.

EXERCISE

Choose a past trauma or grievance. Even if you have not yet achieved empathy, write as though you have. Write from a higher plane than that of judging the one who wronged you or others. Write from the perspective of empathy and compassion.

Remember always that the way we think creates our feelings. The way we feel creates perspective, and our perspective influences outer events. Be aware of what you carry within for it may project outward.

Growth Is Integration

Integration is not possible without growth. One day it dawns on us that the real purpose of the outer life is to serve the inner life's growth toward integration and wholeness. The further and deeper the journey takes us, the more content and inwardly quiet we become. Merging of outer and inner follow so that work and play, mind and body, personal and collective become One.

> *The master in the art of living makes*
> *little distinction*
> *between her work and her play,*
> *her labor and her leisure,*
> *her mind and her body,*
> *her information and her recreation,*
> *her love and her religion.*
> *She hardly knows which is which.*
> *She simply pursues her vision of excellence*
> *at whatever she does, leaving others to*
> *decide whether she is working or playing.*
> *To her, she is always doing both.*
>   Lawrence Pearsall Jacks

Learning to Be Comfortable in the Unknown

Learning to be comfortable in the unknown, with not knowing, is an integral part of the inner journey. This does not mean that you always know what is going to happen. You can move forward even in the state of unknowing, trusting the inner process that when it is time to know, knowing will come. The invisibles will be there to light the way. Meanwhile, even if all is not yet clear, muster the courage to remain in uncertainty while trusting the inner process.

Many years ago, I was in the middle of an acting engagement where I was playing the female lead in a revival of an old Sidney Kingsley play, *The Patriots*. After the stage run of the Pulitzer Prize–winning play, *Great Performances* decided to film it for PBS television. Even though this was all very good, something had changed in me during the run of the show, and I knew it was time to stop acting. There was no outer reason, only a clear inner feeling. So trusting this inner voice, I finished the stage and television job, and then simply stopped acting. There was a three-month period where I had no idea what was next. I meditated and trusted that when it was time to know, knowing would come.

Then I was invited to be a bridesmaid at a friend's wedding just outside of New York City and to spend the weekend there with the couple and their close friends. Among the guests was an astrologer whom I had never met. As we had time, he offered to look at my chart. Knowing nothing about me or what livelihood I had, he told me that he saw an acting career but that writing would be much more important. Writing was my true vocation in this life. I laughed and realized that somehow I had known this all along as I had always written but had never considered it as a possible livelihood. He said I would do even better as a writer. Gratefully, I took this advice and never looked back. As I waited and trusted, an ally appeared to guide. Later, too, I realized how my years as an actor were invaluable in order to later write plays and movies. When asked if I miss acting, I say, "No, the difference now is that I play all the roles as I create them." All the parts of one's life make sense in retrospect.

The Bliss of Not Knowing

I smile when I remember that I became much happier in my life when I realized that I don't know and I don't need to know. Something greater knows.

Sometimes the danger of an inner awakening — no matter how deep and true — is the illusion that the work is done. After years of spiritual work in India, I once naively believed that understanding was complete, that I did know, and that this knowing would safeguard me from the uncertainties of life. Not so. Life *is* uncertainty. Life is change. Life is growth. So I came to accept that I did not know. However, I came to trust that I would be shown all that was needed for my journey. The twist is that once I surrendered "knowing," I was free to enjoy what life presented — moment by moment. And I learned to trust more and more the process of life — not passively but with a deeper awareness.

You can't connect the dots looking forward;
you can only connect them looking backwards.
So you have to trust that the dots will somehow
connect in your future. You have to trust in
something — your gut, destiny, life, karma,
whatever. This approach has never let me down,
and it has made all the difference in my life.

Steve Jobs

Moving Forward

It is time to go forward with our dreams and resolve for a new life, taking with us the lessons from the past. Goals may vary with different individuals, so please take sufficient time with the following ritual. Remember that what matters here is the intention, not just the outer ritual. It is always the intention that gives meaning and power to the ritual.

EXERCISE

- Build a simple altar.

- Place a candle, add something from nature, and a few tokens that have meaning for you and will serve as a focusing tool. This might be a photograph of you as a child or one of parents, grandparents, or a mentor or loved one, as well as special objects that give meaning to your life.

- Place also on the altar an object that symbolizes the future you wish to have.

You have placed some object on the altar that symbolizes "going forward." This may be an intention for you or for the collective. For instance, a painting or statue of a dove to symbolize peace might be placed in the spirit of peace for all. I sometimes put a large feather symbolizing for me a writing quill. Remember that what we think or imagine today can become tomorrow's reality.

EXERCISE

- Sit quietly with closed eyes, and ask yourself, "What needs to be released in order to move forward?"

- You might wish to write it down on a small piece of paper and place it on your altar. All that matters is to take a firm resolve as you do so.

- "I am ready to release _____ so that my journey may continue without obstacles."

By focused journaling and a firm commitment from your heart to heal your own dark residues, you can acquire a lifelong habit of choosing the stories and thoughts that feed the loving, compassionate wolf that lives within (as illustrated in the Introduction). Contribute to the collective by feeding the stories and thoughts that heal.

In this way, global healing takes place one individual, one tribe at a time.

EXERCISE

- Close your eyes. Be still for a moment.

- Then ask yourself this question: "What does it mean to have a life of one's own?"

- When you are ready, write down what comes. Be as specific as possible.

EXERCISE

- Breathe deeply, focusing on the area between the heart and solar plexus.

- Close your eyes, breathe from this center, and ask for the healing that you need. It is more than all right to ask for what we need. Be aware of what rises within. Images. Thoughts. Feelings.

- Write them all down.

EXERCISE

- Imagine it is the end of your life. Imagine all the things you regret not having said or done.

- Your list of what you might regret not doing is a window into what can give your life meaning now.

- What would you have liked to say to a loved one? Write it down.

- What opportunity do you wish you had taken?
  Write it down.

It accomplishes little to give time to blaming yourself or others. Who can say what mistakes are needed in order for the soul to grow? No judgment is needed here. Life is a river that keeps flowing and changing its course at the proper time. Life is also cyclical. Often one life must end before the new one may begin. Are you holding on to a life that no longer serves? Is it time for a change? It is easy to fall into the error of holding tightly to the life whose time has ended. This might be the end of a marriage, the death of a loved one, the end of a career, a child leaving the nest. In another light, these happenings can be seen as an opportunity of a new life calling you. Resistance only delays the new. Remember that you have a choice. Remember, also, that nothing happens until you decide. Such a crossroad is a place of power and potential.

EXERCISE

You stand at a crossroads in your life. From where you are standing, three options are possible. You can go backward, forward, or simply stay where you are.

- First, take a step backward and visualize what this would mean in your life. Write it down.

- Now, take a step forward, and visualize what that might be. Write it down.

- Finally, simply stay where you are going neither back nor forward, and imagine what that would feel like. Write it down.

- Now take a moment and choose which of the three options feels right for now.

- Commit to whatever choice you have made today. Write it down, beginning with "I commit to _____."

EXERCISE

———

- Now imagine that you are at the end of your life, only this time you have done all you had ever wished to do.

- How does it feel?

- Now close your eyes and imagine the happiest moment in your life. What has given you the most satisfaction and contentment? Write this down as well.

- Now you are back where you started, that is, today. What we most value in life is what gives us meaning. What provides the most meaning for you today? Now is the time to choose. Write this down.

By visualizing what you would like your future to look like, you lay the groundwork for things to come. Remember that there is no action without choice. Remember, too, that for anything to happen, a clear intention must exist in the present.

I want to be a soaring gull that leaves no tracks in the sand or sky in its journey. I know that what I wish for demands an active waiting, and that when guidance comes, it will arrive at its own time — not mine.

Focused journaling can be a positive tool allowing us to delve deeper and deeper into the journey of Self. We actively wait for guidance, trusting that what is to be known will be shown at the right time. We walk through life turning inward, trusting not the transient world but something greater than our limited ego.

Healing is the way toward integration and wholeness. This is what some call *spirituality*. Life is a journey toward wholeness. It is nothing less than the soul's journey home.

EXERCISE

- What world do you wish to create? Describe this world.

- Accept responsibility for your creation so that global healing may begin now — one person at a time.

The Bliss of Not Knowing

I actually have a bumper sticker on my car that reads, "Something wonderful is about to happen." Always believe that something wonderful is about to happen. Life is a journey, an incredible journey. With clarity of intention and the space for something new to come, life's journey is full of possibility.

Now and then it's good to pause in our
pursuit of happiness and just be happy.
Guillaume Apollinaire

EXERCISE

• At the sacred altar you earlier created, prepare now for the closing ritual.

• Light the candle.

• Meditate for a few moments. Feel free to add or change anything you like to the words below. Then, say these words — or any of your choosing — aloud:

"I ask for clarity of direction, a new creative vision, serving the collective as a writer and teacher.

May I connect and work with those well suited to a greater purpose.

May old projects be revived and new ones commence.

I let go now of outworn emotional patterns which no longer serve.

May I join with kindred souls and work for the good of all sentient beings.

To this end, I commit my body, mind, and spirit."

A great householder Sage in south India once said to me, "How can you fear the world when it is one you create at each and every moment?"

> *In the immensity of consciousness,*
> *a light appears — a tiny point which*
> *moves rapidly and traces shapes, thoughts,*
> *and feelings, like a pen writing on paper.*
> *And the ink which leaves a trace is memory.*
> *You are that tiny point and by your*
> *movement the world is ever re-created.*
>   Sri Nisargadatta, *I Am That*

Parting Words

Throughout this book, you have learned that it is possible to re-vision your life. You have embraced and integrated the opposites that live within us all, and experienced standing in the light while facing the dark. You have acquired new tools of dialoguing with the soul and other focused journaling techniques. You have traveled a shamanic journey and communicated with spirit and ancestral guides that will continue to walk by your side. You have transcended the archetype of your birth by exploring and expanding your own personal myth. Further, you have learned that trauma can be overcome with imagination by going beyond traditional psychology. And finally you have looked back and integrated the lessons of the past in order to grow forward.

Perhaps some will wish to return to this book as a practice or form a group to work together doing the exercises, then sharing what arises. Discover how your growth will find different responses every time.

Remember always that the solution to any challenge lies within and all that is needed rests dormant, waiting for you to tap into infinite wisdom. Know, too, that you are the creator of your world.

> *Watch your thoughts, they become words.*
> *Watch your words, they become actions.*
> *Watch your actions, they become habits.*
> *Watch your habits, they become character.*
> *Watch your character, it becomes your destiny.*
> Lao Tzu

From Rumi, the thirteenth-century Persian mystic and poet, I leave you with the following invocation:

> *No more words. Hear only the voice within.*
> Rumi

Also by
Catherine Ann Jones

TELEVISION
Child of Destiny (Last Queen of Hawaii)
It's Only Women (The Dalkon Shield Scandal)
Death of an Innocent Child (starring Ellen Burstyn)
Summertime
Touched by an Angel (series)

FILM & CABLE
The Pact
Sammy and Son
Wolfbride
Poe: The Dark Angel
The Christmas Wife (starring Jason Robards, Julie Harris)
Unlikely Angel (starring Dolly Parton)
Angel Passing (co-writer), (starring Hume Cronyn,
    Calista Flockhart)

PLAYS
Calamity Jane
Calamity and Wild Bill the musical
The Women of Cedar Creek
The Myth of Annie Beckman
On the Edge: The Final Years of Virginia Woolf
Somewhere-in-Between
Difficult Friends

The Hill
The Friend
A Fairytale for Adults

HONORS FOR WRITING
National Endowment for the Arts for Best Play
Winner of 15 awards at film festivals, both US and abroad
Emmy-nominated for Best Film, Best Writing
Ludwig Vogelstein Award
Asian Council, John D. Rockefeller III Grant for Research
Beverly Hills Theatre Guild/Julie Harris Award
New York Drama League for Best Play
Fulbright-Hays Research Scholar
CIIS Distinguished Visitor to India
Yaddo Foundation
MacDowell Foundation
Wurlitzer Foundation
Aspen Playwrights Award
Eugene O'Neill Playwrights Conference
National Merit Scholar

PROFESSIONAL AFFLIATIONS/TEACHING
Pacifica Graduate Institute, MA, Mythology & Depth
    Psychology; faculty
University of Texas, BFA, Theatre Arts; faculty
Actors Studio (NYC) Playwrights-Directors Unit;
    HB Studio (NYC); faculty
Dramatist Guild, PEN, WGA, SAG, AFTRA, AEA,
    Academy of Television Arts & Sciences
The New School University (NYC) — Playwriting
    faculty, seven years

University of Southern California (LA) Graduate Film/
    Screenwriting — faculty, six years; Columbia
    University, Skidmore College, National Film
    School of Greece, British Film Institute (London),
    British Arts Council, National Drama School/
    India, Film School/Indonesia; Esalen Institute,
    Omega Institute, Kripalu, Krotona Institute, etc.

PUBLICATIONS
The Way of Story: The Craft & Soul of Writing
    (Michael Wiese Productions, 2007)
Confrontation; El Dorado Sun; W.B. Yeats Society;
    Ojai Valley News; American Vendantist

About the Author

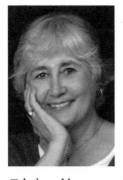 CATHERINE ANN JONES holds a graduate degree in Depth Psychology and Archetypal Mythology from Pacifica Graduate Institute where she has also taught. After playing major roles in over fifty plays, she became disappointed by the lack of good roles for women and wrote a play about Virginia Woolf (*On the Edge*) and her struggle with madness in a world gone mad, i.e., WWII. The play won a National Endowment for the Arts Award. Ten of her plays, including *Calamity Jane* (both play and musical) and *The Women of Cedar Creek*, have won multiple awards and are produced both in and out of New York. Her films include *The Christmas Wife* (starring Jason Robards and Julie Harris), *Unlikely Angel* (starring Dolly Parton), and the popular TV series, *Touched by an Angel*. A Fulbright Research Scholar to India studying shamanism, she has taught at The New School University, University of Southern California, Pacifica Graduate Institute, and the Esalen and the Omega Institutes. Her book, *The Way of Story: The Craft & Soul of Writing*, is used in many schools, including New York University writing programs. Ms. Jones lives in Ojai, California, and leads workshops throughout the United States, Europe, and Asia. For online courses, blog, workshops, and writing consultant services please visit *www.wayofstory.com*.

HERE ARE OTHER **DIVINE ARTS** BOOKS YOU MAY ENJOY

THE SACRED SITES OF THE DALAI LAMAS

by Glenn H. Mullin

"As this most beautiful book reveals, the Dalai Lamas continue to teach us that there are, indeed, other ways of thinking, other ways of being, other ways of orienting ourselves in social, spiritual, and ecological space."

— Wade Davis, Explorer-in-Residence, National Geographic Society

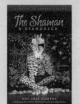

THE SHAMAN & AYAHUASCA: *Journeys to Sacred Realms*

by Don José Campos

"This remarkable and beautiful book suggests a path back to understanding the profound healing and spiritual powers that are here for us in the plant world. This extraordinary book shows a way toward reawakening our respect for the natural world, and thus for ourselves."

— John Robbins, author, *The Food Revolution* and *Diet for a New America*

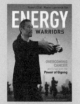

ENERGY WARRIORS
Overcoming Cancer and Crisis with the Power of Qigong

by Bob Ellal and Lawrence Tan

"The combination of Ellal's extraordinary true story and Master Tan's depth of knowledge about the relationship between martial arts and wellness makes for a unique and important contribution to the growing body of literature about holistic thinking and living."

— Jean Benedict Raffa, author, *Healing the Sacred Divide* and *The Bridge to Wholeness*

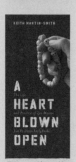

A HEART BLOWN OPEN:
The Life & Practice of Zen Master Jun Po Denis Kelly Roshi

by Keith Martin-Smith

"This is the story of our time... an absolute must-read for anyone with even a passing interest in human evolution..."

— Ken Wilber, author, *Integral Spirituality*

"This is the legendary story of an inspiring teacher that mirrors the journey of many contemporary Western seekers."

— Alex Grey, artist and author of *Transfigurations*

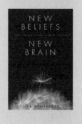

NEW BELIEFS NEW BRAIN:
Free Yourself from Stress and Fear

by Lisa Wimberger

"Lisa Wimberger has earned the right, through trial by fire, to be regarded as a rising star among meditation teachers. No matter where you are in your journey, *New Beliefs, New Brain* will shine a light on your path."

— Marianne Williamson, author, *A Return to Love* and *Everyday Grace*

YEAR ZERO: *Time of the Great Shift*

by Kiara Windrider

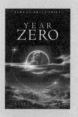

"I can barely contain myself as I implode with gratitude for the gift of *Year Zero*! Every word resonates on a cellular level, awakening ancient memories and realigning my consciousness with an unshakable knowing that the best has yet to come. This is more than a book; it is a manual for building the new world!"

— Mikki Willis, founder, ELEVATE

ILAHINOOR: *Awakening the Divine Human*

by Kiara Windrider

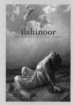

"Ilahinoor is a truly precious and powerful gift for those yearning to receive and integrate Kiara Windrider's guidance on their journey for spiritual awakening and wisdom surrounding the planet's shifting process."

— Alexandra Delis-Abrams, Ph.D., author *Attitudes, Beliefs, and Choices*

THE MESSAGE: *A Guide to Being Human*

by LD Thompson

"Simple, profound, and moving! The author has been given a gift... a beautiful way to distill the essence of life into an easy-to-read set of truths, with wonderful examples along the way. Listen... for that is how it all starts."

— Lee Carroll, author, the *Kryon* series; co-author, *The Indigo Children*

SOPHIA—THE FEMININE FACE OF GOD:
Nine Heart Paths to Healing and Abundance

by Karen Speerstra

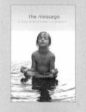

"Karen Speerstra shows us most compellingly that when we open our hearts, we discover the wisdom of the Feminine all around us. A totally refreshing exploration, and beautifully researched read."

— Michael Cecil, author, *Living at the Heart of Creation*

A FULLER VIEW: *Buckminster Fuller's Vision of Hope and Abundance for All*

by L. Steven Sieden

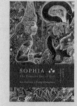

"This book elucidates Buckminster Fuller's thinking, honors his spirit, and creates an enthusiasm for continuing his work."

— Marianne Williamson, author, *Return To Love* and *Healing the Soul of America*

GAIA CALLS: *South Sea Voices, Dolphins, Sharks & Rainforests*

by Wade Daok

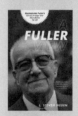

"Wade has the soul of a dolphin, and has spent a life on and under the oceans on a quest for deep knowledge. This is an important book that will change our views of the ocean and our human purpose."

— Ric O'Barry, author, *Behind the Dolphin Smile* and star of *The Cove,* which won the 2010 Academy Award for Best Documentary

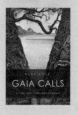

1.800.833.5738 • 25% discount available online • www.divineartsmedia.com

Divine Arts sprang to life fully formed
as an intention to bring spiritual practice
into daily life.

*Human beings are far more than the one-dimensional creatures perceived
by most of humanity and held static in consensus reality. There is a deep
and vast body of knowledge — both ancient and emerging — that informs
and gives us the understanding, through direct experience, that we are
magnificent creatures occupying many dimensions with untold powers and
connectedness to all that is.*

*Divine Arts books and films explore these realms, powers, and teachings
through inspiring, informative, and empowering works by pioneers,
artists, and great teachers from all the wisdom traditions. We invite your
participation and look forward to learning how we may serve you.*

Onward and upward,
Michael Wiese, Publisher

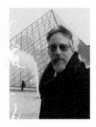